SIMPLE METHODS FOR WOMEN'S GUT HEALTH THAT WORK

TIPS AND TRICKS TO IMPROVE DIGESTION, RESTORE YOUR HEALTH & RECHARGE YOUR BODY AND MIND

ELLA RENÉE

A GIFT TO MY READERS

Please enjoy your own copy of my 10-Day Weight Loss Challenge!

Included in your 10-day challenge is a weight loss meal plan, at home or in the gym exercise program, and daily life-changing habits for long-term weight loss success.

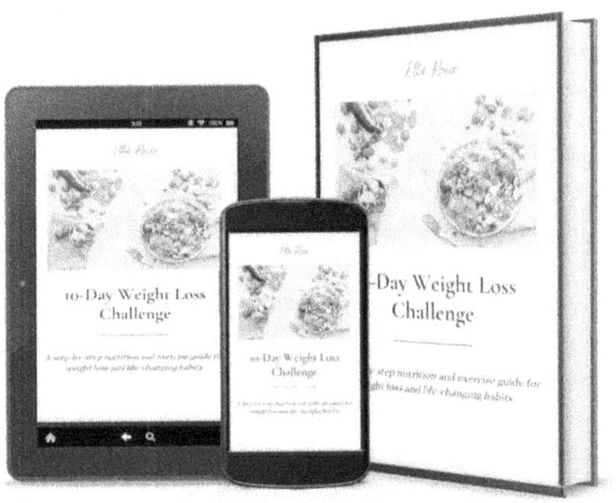

Scan the QR code to download your FREE copy today!

CONTENTS

Introduction 9

Part I
IMPROVE DIGESTION

1. GUT MICROBIOME: THE GUT GARDEN 17
Your Gut Microbiome: The Hidden World 18
Gut Bacteria: Helpful vs. Harmful 21
Fortifying Defenses 22
IBS and Dysbiosis: The Uncooperative Jerks 31
Alleviating the Symptoms of IBS 32
Good Gut Health Practices 36

2. EXERCISE: OPTIMIZING DIGESTION 39
Backed Up? Understanding Healthy Digestion 40
Exercise & Digestion: Cause and Effect 42
Let's Move It - Got Guts? 47
Exercise: Practical Practices 50
Exercises For Better Gut Health 56
Exercise Plan: 10, 30, 60 81

3. MADE IN THE KITCHEN: 30-DAY FLAT TUMMY MEAL PLAN 85
Dieting for Gut Health 86
How To Manage Common Digestive Disorders 89
Your 30-Day Meal Plan for a Flatter Tummy 95

Part II

RESTORE YOUR HEALTH

4. MEET THE ESTROBOLOME: UNDERSTANDING GUT HEALTH AND HORMONES 145
Metabolizing Estrogen: Meet Estrobolome 146
Why Estrogen? 149
Estrobolome and Gut Health 152
Gut Health and Hormonal Balance 154
Healthy Hormones 157

5. FOOD AS A TIME MACHINE: EATING YOUR WAY TO A YOUNGER YOU 161
What's Your Real Age? 162
Healthy Aging 167
Managing Your Biological Age With Food 169
What Are Telomeres? And what do they have to do with aging? 170
Fighting Inflammaging 173
De-Stress Diaries 175
Journaling 178

6. HACKED: 15 TIPS & TRICKS TO KEEPING YOUR GUT HEALTHY 183
1. Don't wait, hydrate! 186
2. Lights Out 187
3. Eat the Rainbow 188
4. Keep Moving 188
5. Keep Away the Sweet Poison 189
6. Tea Time! 190
7. Let's Decaffeinate! 190
8. Probiotics are Your New BFF 191
9. Fill Up on Fruits and Fiber 191
10. Chew Like a Sloth 192
11. Fermented Foods are Fun 192
12. Less Stress is Always Best 192

13. Apple Cider Vinegar for the Win! 193
14. The Bone Broth Secret 194
15. Mindfulness Matters 194

Part III

RECHARGE YOUR MIND & BODY

7. ENS: THE GUT-BRAIN CONNECTION 199
The Gut-Brain Axis: A Beneficial Relationship 200
The Enteric Nervous System: A Two-Way Street 204
The Gut Affects the Brain … And Vice-Versa 206
Gut Health & Mental Health 208
Let's Talk Lifestyle 208

8. MODULATED: MANAGING YOUR MOOD WITH FOOD 211
Are You Really "Hangry"? 212
Here's Why You Calm Down Once You've Eaten Something 214
Using Food to Manage Mood 216
Eat This, Not That 217

Conclusion 223
Bibliography 229

INTRODUCTION

> *"Nourishing yourself in a way that helps you blossom in the direction you want to go is attainable, and you are worth the effort."*
>
> — DEBORAH DAY

Picture this. You wake up bursting with the energy of a Greek goddess. Your skin is glowing, and your hair is so luxurious, so magnificent, that it's swaying perfectly, as though you are in a shampoo commercial! Your mind is reeling with nothing but clarity. It's like you are floating on a calm, blue Caribbean ocean, the sun up ahead basking, giving you life and renewing all your brain cells. You are pumped and ready to go!

Then, suddenly, you find yourself at the gym, on the treadmill. You're working out on high intensity, your luxurious shiny hair bouncing up and down with each step. You feel no pain, your skin is dewy (because Greek goddesses don't sweat), and your abs are as defined as those of an Amazonian warrior. You have finally achieved the dream body you always desired, and your health is finally on track, as you've always wanted. You are living your best life.

At this point, you probably want to ask me if I'm a little tipsy. Or, you want to tell me to stop wasting my time, making you dream impossible dreams. You've been there many times, hoping that, if you just dreamed the impossible dream and did what you were told, you could finally tap into your inner goddess and reach your optimal level of health and fineness.

OK, sure. Perhaps you will never have the chiseled abs of an Amazonian warrior. That takes a dedication, commitment, and time investment that most of us non-Amazonians don't have. But why can't a girl still dream of a flat stomach and a healthy body? We might not be Greek goddesses, but is it too much to ask to want to wear a cute bikini on the beach and feel sexy in it?

What if I told you there is a way to tap into your inner goddess through your gut health? What if there is a way to benefit your entire physical, emotional, and mental health by simply focusing on what you eat and drink? It really is that simple. There is no need for fad diets, 1,000 situps at the gym every day, or starving yourself. You can be healthy, look great, feel great and still enjoy one of life's simplest pleasures: delicious food.

As women, our health is often not prioritized. There is an expectation that we need to look perfect at all times, with 10% body fat, the skin and hair of a supermodel and the abs of a woman who's never eaten a plate of pasta in her life. Nobody really cares whether we are healthy from the inside out. The emphasis is always on looking perfect from the outside alone, whether or not we are actually healthy. To make matters worse, even when we know that there is something wrong with our health; even when we wake up lethargic, or we're unable to sleep because of gastric issues, we're not taken seriously by family, friends, and even doctors. We're simply just blamed and shamed. Like you, and like me, every woman understands the humiliation of being dismissed and mocked when we try to speak out about our health and our bodies. I believe it's time we take back our power and change the way society approaches women's bodies and health. I think it's time we start advocating for ourselves. What better way to begin advocating for ourselves than with you and with me?

As a certified fitness and nutrition coach with hundreds of female clients, I can testify that it is an uphill battle for many of my clients who want to achieve a healthy, balanced lifestyle, but are discouraged at every step. That's why I approach my job with the emotional intelligence, care, comfort, and support that women need to change their lifestyles for the better. Many of my clients are health-seekers who decided to seek professional help one last time before giving up on achieving good health. They have tried every diet but, in the end, always find them to be unsustainable, too expensive, taking up too much of their already busy schedule and leaving them looking and feeling worse than when they started. They have come to realize that most of what is advertised as "healthy" for women, such as fad diets and crash diets, are only exaggerations aimed at making profits for big companies.

If you're reading this book, then you connect with this feeling of constant failure. Every time you try to reach your health goals, you inevitably fail. So, like any intelligent woman, you've decided to try a more natural, holistic approach towards looking and feeling good from the inside out. Don't get me wrong, there's nothing wrong with a woman who wants to look good. However, rather than using plasters to fix deep structural damage, you want to dig through to the root of your health, starting from the foundation upwards. You understand that being healthy and feeling great starts from within, and no amount of specially-formulated lotion with organic, free-range mermaid dust will do that for you. So, naturally, you've come to a compassionate expert to help you successfully eat your way into better health and wellness.

In this book, I'm going to teach you how to change the way your entire body works, by changing how you eat. I'm going to teach you the radical scientific principle that our guts are a "second brain" and how, by keeping your gut healthy, you can keep your entire body healthy too. I will empower you to change your mindset towards your health, rather than simply flitting from one diet to another. With the tools I provide in this book, you will lay the foundation for nourishing and nurturing your gut health using scientifically-approved, easy-to-implement methods and treatments.

Think of me as your personal trainer and nutritionist. To help you along the way on your journey to gut health, I have compiled some of my favorite, most gut-healthy easy-to-make recipes, as well as practical approaches for keeping your gut in tip-top condition! I have also packed this book with beginner-friendly gut-optimizing lifestyle choices so that you too can wake up bursting with energy and boasting a clear mind and flat stomach. Even better, they can all be easily incorporated into your daily schedule and rituals, so there is no need to waste money and precious time trying to change your life to fit a new lifestyle. Instead, you can let your new lifestyle work for you!

So grab your hair brush, your string bikini, and your organic, free-range mermaid dust lotion, and let's get gut healthy!

PART I

IMPROVE DIGESTION

1

GUT MICROBIOME: THE GUT GARDEN

> *"Take care of your body. It's the only place you have to live."*
>
> — JIM ROHN

Did you know that we each have roughly 100 trillion bacteria living in and around our bodies at all times? I like to think of these bacteria as organisms living on a planet: Planet Me. Their astronauts are studying their world, me, just as humans study planet Earth. These bacteria are in an existential crisis, trying to decipher where they came from and if there are other planets (and other bacterial life forms) out there. It's a silly idea, but I love it! And who's to say it's not true? Who's to say, one day, they won't make contact with other bacterial life forms on other human planets? Or, maybe my dad was right, and I have an overactive imagination?

Whether my dad was right or not (he was), your planet is hospitable to your gut microbiome, just as Earth is hospitable to us humans. And, just as Earth provides us with the perfect conditions that allow us to thrive and to reproduce, our guts provide our bacteria with the perfect conditions for thriving and multiplying.

In this chapter, we will discuss the gut microbiome, notably what it is and why it is so crucial to our gut health and digestion. We will also discuss the health benefits available to you when you cultivate a healthy gut microbiome.

YOUR GUT MICROBIOME: THE HIDDEN WORLD

The first time I heard of the gut microbiome, I was honestly put off. In all fairness, I was still an immature teenager, but you have to admit, the thought of having 100 trillion bacteria living inside of and on you isn't exactly appealing. If it were, you would have added it to your dating profile by now.

"Single, fun-loving bacteria-packed woman seeking a man with at least 200 trillion bacteria in his gut."

Yuck!

Ironically, while gut bacteria is decidedly not sexy, it is what makes us look sexy from the inside out. In that case, boasting about your bacteria-packed status is actually accurate and I wildly encourage you to use it on your own dating profile.

Let's say you take my advice (naturally), and you match with an equally sexy, attractive man. He takes you on a date to a four-star restaurant with the best shrimp you have ever had, and he asks you what exactly your gut microbiome is and why it is so important that you added it to your dating profile. Don't you worry! I'm about to teach you what it is, so you will always have sexy dating conversation starters!

Put simply, your gut microbiome is made up of the trillions of bacteria, parasites, fungi, viruses, and other microorganisms in your gut that work to ensure your body's day-to-day functions run smoothly. These microorganisms, also known as microbiomes, microbiota, and microflora of the gut, live mostly in our guts, although some live in other parts of the human body, like the mouth (oral microbes), the skin (skin microbes), and the reproductive system (reproductive microbes).

Most of them are friendly, meaning they are beneficial for your health. However, some can be potentially harmful and pathogenic, causing serious illnesses.

Both healthy and pathogenic microorganisms live pretty peacefully with each other on Planet You. But, Planet You is a very fragile place. The smallest changes can disrupt the lives of your microbe civilization. Just like on planet Earth! Changes like using antibiotics, a change in your diet, or infections can disrupt your microbiome's peace.

Your gut microbiome's main job is to help you digest your food, although scientists believe they also support your heart health, the health of your central nervous system (which contributes to brain health) and a healthy immune system. I think it's pretty interesting that everyone has their own unique colony of microbiota in their gut, determined by their DNA, diet, environment, and the microorganisms you are introduced to when you are born. The next time someone tries to tell you that you're not unique, or you're too basic, you can use this fun fact against them.

Your microbes (of which there are up to 1,000 species) are mostly found in your large intestine, in a pocket called your "cecum," and others are found in your small intestine. Many of these species are also responsible for digesting fiber, which is a very important part of your health, helping to prevent diabetes, heart disease, cancer, and weight gain.

At this point of your evening, your date is now leaning in towards you, his eyes sparkling with wonder that a woman as gorgeous as you knows so much information about the bacteria that live in our guts. He wants to know more! Well, buckle in, because you're about to learn more hidden tips for making a man (or woman) fall wildly in love with your unrivaled sophistication!

GUT BACTERIA: HELPFUL VS. HARMFUL

A healthy gut bacteria balance makes you feel energetic and happy, promoting good physical health and mental health. They break down potentially toxic food compounds, help you absorb nutrients, boost your immune system, and prevent unhealthy bacteria from causing infections. It's an all-out turf war in your gut, where your good and bad bacteria break into Grease-like dance numbers whenever they encounter each other, each outdancing the other in flamboyant ways, to claim victory over your intestines. As your healthy bacteria dances, twirls, and spins, it promotes good HDL cholesterol and triglycerides, two things your heart needs to be healthy. It also produces short-chain fatty acids (SCFA), which your body uses as a nutrient source. SCFAs also improve your muscle function and prevent chronic diseases, including bowel disorders, and some types of cancers.

The more you feed your healthy gut microbe with good food, the more energy they have to practice their dance moves and reproduce. And, here's the plus. Not only will the right foods cultivate good conditions for your gut microflora, but other lifestyle factors, such as regular exercise, low stress levels, plenty of sleep, and avoiding antibiotics, also help.

An unhealthy gut microbiota balance (also known as gut microbiota dysbiosis), on the other hand, can lead to serious health complications, such as obesity, cancer, cardiovascular diseases, metabolic disease, leaky gut syndrome, inflammatory bowel disease, gastrointestinal disorders, allergy-related diseases, and central nervous system related diseases. These guys are really bad to the bone!

FORTIFYING DEFENSES

You are lying in the shade on a beautiful beach. The sun is high in the sky, making your entire body feel like a warm cinnamon donut. The sea is a beautiful, serene blue, swishing away all your anxiety. The bar staff hands you another chilled mimosa, as you settle in to read your favorite book. It is perfection - No! Heaven!

The same way you have dreams of the perfect environment is the same way your microbiome dreams of its perfect environment. In your dream environment, you are happy, thriving, glowing, and maybe even smelling like a freshly-baked cinnamon roll, i.e., delicious. In your microbiome's dream environment, they are also happy, thriving, and… well, maybe not glowing, since they have no skin. And maybe not smelling good since they do live in the intestines. Anyway, as I was saying, you cannot glow if they are not digesting! So, it's in your best interest to create an environment as close to their ideal as possible. That way, they will become strong enough and relaxed enough to do their job, fighting off bad flora and keeping your entire body healthy. Here's how.

The Good

In order to promote good bacteria in your gut follow this advice:

- Eat a diverse diet rich in whole foods

The more diverse your diet is, the more species of bacteria will be able to survive in your intestines.

If you want to eat a diverse diet, you will need to cut out the traditional Western diet from your palette. It is too high in fat, sugar, and processed foods to feed your microflora. Put the strawberry cheesecake down and make yourself a strawberry smoothie instead!

- Eat fermented foods

Fermented foods are usually rich in a bacteria known as Lactobacilli. People who eat a lot of yogurt, for example, have a gut rich in Lactobacilli, but also less of the bad bacteria known as Enterobacteriaceae.

Yogurt is one of the most popular fermented foods because it is versatile, readily available, and cheap. If you choose to incorporate yogurt into your diet, go for plain, unsweetened yogurt made out of milk and bacteria mixtures (which are called "live active cultures") on the label. Other wonderful fermented foods that you can incorporate into your diet include kombucha, sauerkraut, kimchi, kefir, and tempeh.

- Eat whole grains

Whole grains contain insoluble fiber, a type of carb that cannot be absorbed by the small intestine. As a result, they move onto the large intestine where they enable beneficial bacteria, such as Bifidobacteria, Lactobacilli, and Bacteroidetes to grow. You may have heard people talk about how they "add bulk to your bowel movements," and, more than likely, you may have experienced this classy phenomenon too. Whole grains are great at increasing your feelings of fullness, preventing you from overeating. That's why a plate of brown rice is more filling than the same plate of white rice. However, if you have celiac disease or a gluten sensitivity, then you should avoid whole grains that contain gluten because it leads to intestinal permeability (which is when material begins to pass from inside of your gastrointestinal tract into the rest of your body, sometimes causing leaky gut syndrome).

- Eat plenty of beans, legumes, fruits, and vegetables

If your parents ever complained that you don't eat enough fruit and vegetables, then they were right, and you need to apologize to them. Fruits, vegetables, legumes, and beans are the best sources of nutrients available for our gut health. They prevent disease-causing bacteria from growing in your intestines and are high in fiber, which feeds some of the healthy bacteria in your gut.

- Eat polyphenol-rich foods

Polyphenols are very healthy plant compounds that reduce inflammation, bad cholesterol levels, blood pressure, and oxidative stress. Polyphenol-rich foods include green tea, almonds, onions, blueberries, red wine, grape skins, broccoli, and cocoa. Cocoa and red wine have been shown to increase the amount of Lactobacilli and Bifidobacteria, while reducing the amount of unhealthy bacteria, Clostridia.

- Eat prebiotic foods

Prebiotic foods are mainly made up of insoluble fiber and complex carbs that human cells are unable to digest. Your body sends them to the large intestine to be digested instead. Prebiotic-rich foods include fruits, legumes, and vegetables. Introduce prebiotic food to your diet gradually, otherwise, it could cause gas and bloating. Sure, you might be really healthy if you eat a big bowl of chili for lunch, then follow that with a big bowl of raw cabbage for dinner. However, people may not want to sit next to you in the office if you do.

- Consume probiotics

Probiotics are live microorganisms, just like the microorganisms in your gut. These temporary residents are usually bacteria or yeast and will stay in your gut for just a little while after you ingest them. However, they are powerful enough to clean up your gut while in there, leaving the whole place healthy and nourished. Fermented foods are probiotic-rich. Alternatively, you can take probiotic supplements.

- Eat plenty of plants

Research has shown that a vegetarian diet is healthier than an omnivorous diet because they are richer in fiber and nutrients. Not to say you can't be just as healthy as a vegetarian. You just need to step up your veggie game. Make sure there are plenty of colorful vegetables alongside your free-range chicken.

The Bad

Some bad bacteria, such as Clostridium difficile, already naturally live in your gut. However, they live in such a small amount that they can't really do any harm to you. Other common ways that bad bacteria get into your body are of course, eating contaminated food or not washing your hands regularly. Seriously, don't be that person not washing your hands after coming out of the washroom. It's not cool, and you could end up contaminating your body with bad bacteria. When you ingest contaminated water or food, if you have a healthy gut microbe, they can usually protect you from these pathogenic bacteria.

Then, there is also the problem of taking antibiotics for your health. Antibiotics do not discriminate between healthy-friendly bacteria and pathogenic ones. It kills your healthy bacteria, giving any bad bacteria that survive a chance to rise up and defeat the enemy! Other medications can do the same including, believe it or not, hormonal medicines. It's always best to speak with your doctor before taking any medication.

Signs you have too much bad bacteria include:

- Gaining weight/losing weight
- Sleep disturbance
- Fatigue
- Food allergies/intolerance
- Skin conditions, such as rashes
- Chronic illnesses (as have been discussed in this chapter)

- Constipation/diarrhea
- Abdominal cramps
- Abdominal bloating

The Ugly

Gut Microbiota Dysbiosis is a medical condition that occurs when the unhealthy bacteria in your gut have overcrowded and overpowered the healthy bacteria. You can have a mild case of dysbiosis, such as stomach upset, which your body is actually able to correct on its own without any medication. Other times, medication and lifestyle changes are enough to reverse dysbiosis. If your symptoms are severe and do not improve, it is best to consult a doctor or visit an emergency room.

Causes of dysbiosis include:

- New medication killing off your healthy microbiome.
- Poor dental hygiene, causing your oral microbiota to become unbalanced.
- A weak immune system.
- Being exposed to harmful bacteria.
- Consuming two or more alcoholic drinks daily.
- Consuming chemicals, for example, from pesticides and antibiotics on food.
- Increased sugar intake.

- Increased food additives in your diet.

Having dysbiosis increases your risk of developing the following:

- Irritable Bowel Syndrome (IBS)
- Late-onset dementia
- Parkinson's disease
- Colon/rectal cancer
- Diabetes
- Having trouble thinking/concentrating
- Nausea
- Halitosis (bad breath)
- Anxiety
- Leaky gut syndrome
- Obesity
- Polycystic ovary syndrome (PCOS)
- Candida, a yeast-caused fungi infection
- Skin conditions
- Liver disease
- Celiac disease
- Heart disease/heart failure

IBS AND DYSBIOSIS: THE UNCOOPERATIVE JERKS

IBS (Irritable Bowel Syndrome) and dysbiosis negatively affect digestion by changing our digestive system. Sometimes this change is brought about by dysbiosis, although not always. Like dysbiosis, IBS can cause symptoms such as bloating, constipation, diarrhea, abdominal cramping, excess gas, changes in bowel frequency, changes in stool shape and size, and excessive and sudden weight loss.

If you are experiencing undigested food in your stool, as well as other symptoms discussed in this chapter, then you need to see your doctor because it could be a sign of an overly sensitive colon, causing IBS. Our digestive system is linked so intricately to other parts of our health that emotional problems, such as stress and anxiety, can also lead to IBS. Other lifestyle and environmental factors such as a lack of exercise, are also a cause of IBS.

Although we know the causes of dysbiosis, it's still not clear what exactly causes IBS. In fact, it is also not clear why some things trigger IBS in some people and not others. Nevertheless, common triggers may include:

- Stone fruits, such as mangos and peaches
- Wheat
- Coffee
- Tea
- Certain vegetables, such as broccoli and asparagus
- Dairy products
- Beans
- Artificial sweeteners
- Chocolate

ALLEVIATING THE SYMPTOMS OF IBS

IBS is one of the milder digestive disorders. That's why you can use home remedies to provide relief from cramping, gas, bloating, and diarrhea. At no point in history has anyone ever said, "Wow! I'd like some more diarrhea, please! Thank God I have IBS!" But there have been many curse words thrown out when the symptoms of IBS flare up! Try these home treatments instead. They are much more effective than curse words.

Relax

According to the International Foundation for Functional Gastrointestinal Disorders, these three relaxation techniques are effective for reducing IBS symptoms:

Diaphragmatic/abdominal breathing

Your diaphragm is located above your belly button, just below your ribcage. To proceed with diaphragmatic/abdominal breathing, all you need to do is fill your diaphragm as much as possible. Place your hands above your diaphragm and notice how much air you're breathing in and breathing out. Breathe in slowly, filling the oxygen all the way to the bottom of your abdomen. Your hands will rise as you do. Hold your breath for a few seconds, then slowly breathe out. Repeat 5-10 times. If you feel light-headed, stop and return to normal breath for 20 seconds before starting again.

Progressive muscle relaxation

Lie or sit down in a comfortable place, then take four deep abdominal breaths.

Frown deeply, tensing the muscles in your forehead. Stay in this position for 4 seconds, then release. You will notice your muscles relaxing when you do this.

Move onto your eyelids, squeezing them together for four seconds. Release and open your eyes; notice how the muscles around your eyes are relaxing. You can use muscle relaxation for nearly every muscle in your body. When you are done, take another 40 abdominal breaths, and notice if there are any other muscles in your body that are still tense. If there are, use progressive muscle relaxation on those muscles as well.

Visualization/positive imagery

Settle in a quiet, comfortable place, either lying down or sitting down in a comfortable position. Make sure there are no distractions around you as you close your eyes and begin to imagine yourself in a relaxing, calm, and peaceful environment. This could mean different things for different people. Some people imagine themselves in the middle of the ocean in a boat, while some people imagine themselves in their grandmother's house. Imagine a place that invokes peace and positive emotions within you. Begin to notice all the different things in this place. If you're in the middle of the ocean, notice the clouds up ahead and how blue the sky is. As you breathe in deeply and slowly using abdominal breaths, let your imagination take you away from the present, away from your worries, stress, and anxiety.

Begin to imagine that any pain and discomfort you feel from your digestive disorder is leaving you so that you now feel completely relaxed and free of pain and discomfort. Stay in this place where no pain or discomfort exists for as long as you want to, until you feel completely relaxed, calm, and at peace. Don't worry if you find your mind wandering. This is normal. If that happens, all you need to do is bring yourself back to your focus, to your breath, and to your peaceful place.

Eat your whole grains

What's the point of berating your dates if you don't eat your whole grains regularly? Eat your fiber, girl! It's recommended that you add fiber to your diet gradually. This gives your gut microbiome a chance to get used to it, reducing your chances of IBS' embarrassing symptoms. To make things less awkward, take a fiber supplement instead. There! Problem solved.

Put down the milk

Everyone had that friend in school who was lactose intolerant and still refused to give up dairy. For the sake of the people you love, please just give up dairy. If you absolutely must have dairy, replace recipes that call for milk, cheese, and cream with lactose-free yogurt. If you can't stomach yogurt, then you could try using enzyme supplements that help you break down lactose.

Laxatives are tricky

Try using a laxative, it can be a quick way to solve your problem. Just use laxatives with caution and follow the label instructions closely.

Avoid large quantities of the following foods:

- Cabbage
- Cauliflower
- Chocolate
- Alcohol
- Coffee
- Broccoli
- Soda (even a small amount can cause an issue)

Get off your butt and exercise

Regular exercise is a great way to relieve IBS symptoms. More about this in the next chapter!

GOOD GUT HEALTH PRACTICES

Before you move on, let's look at some tips for your inner enthusiast, so you can begin achieving gut health NOW. Let's be honest, who really likes being patient? We all know it's wrong to want instant gratification, but it feels so right! I personally believe it's OK to feed your inner gratification monster once in a while. It keeps you from pigging out on cheeseburgers and ice cream on those nights when you simply get fed up of being patient and delaying gratification.

In other words, give in to your inner devil with these gut-healthy tips that are not only cost-effective but also practical and easy:

- Go for a brisk 20-minute walk just after waking up or before bed. Eat a banana before your walk to power you with energy and to feed your gut microbe with healthy nutrients.
- Whenever you eat something healthy, picture your microbiota receiving reinforcements in a warzone. I like to make this picture as ridiculous as possible, because not only does it make me laugh and feel good, it reminds me of why I am pursuing a healthier lifestyle. Sometimes I picture the bacteria with military helmets on or with bayonets, ready to attack all the evil pathogens trying to invade my gut. Make the image as ridiculous as possible. Remember that stress only makes your unhealthy bacteria stronger, while laughing and releasing stress sends much-needed reinforcements to your army of bacteria!
- Where a recipe calls for white flour, swap for oat flour. Oat flour easily replaces white flour

in most recipes and is one of your gut microflora's favorite foods.

- Drink a mug of green tea with cinnamon after lunch every day. The best way I can show you how important green tea is for digestion and a flat stomach is by making you do an experiment. I challenge you to drink 2 cups of green tea every day for a week. At the end of the week, take a picture of your stomach from the side angle. Then, forgo the cups of green tea and replace them with water every day for another week. At the end of the second week, compare the differences between the first and second weeks. The difference will be clear. Your stomach will be noticeably flatter at the end of week one.
- Add a few extra cloves of garlic to your meals when cooking them. Garlic is antibacterial and antiviral. It kills harmful bacteria and viruses in your gut without destroying healthy bacteria and viruses.

Your gut microbiome is a part of you, so you should treat them well. If you treat them well, they will treat you well in return.

2

EXERCISE: OPTIMIZING DIGESTION

> *"What seems impossible today will one day become your warm-up."*
>
> — ANONYMOUS

Now that you've completed Chapter One, you know enough about gut health to appreciate the importance of exercise in aiding healthy digestion. Your gut loves exercise. It's as simple as that!

In this chapter, we are going to discover, in more depth, the benefits of exercise in relation to gut health, as well as how to optimize your digestion through regular exercise. Essentially, you know the basics, so in this chapter, we're going to get down to the nitty-gritty of exercise.

In our gym-obsessed, protein shake-obsessed, macros-counting, I never-miss-my-yoga-class-obsessed culture, I think it's easy to feel lost. For women who are new to fitness culture, it can feel as though you are learning an entirely new language or subculture - which you are! When women feel left out, they often opt out of a healthy lifestyle as a result. I don't want you to feel confused or to feel left out of the wonderful benefits of being fit. I also want you to be able to go to your lunch dates with your girlfriends with your yoga mat casually swung on your shoulders so they know how dedicated to your gut health you really are.

So, to give you the spirit and encouragement you need, I have added practical tips on how to incorporate exercise into your day-to-day activities (especially if you have a packed schedule). That means you have no excuse not to exercise and send reinforcements to your gut microflora. As one of my favorite motivational sayings goes: "What seems impossible today will one day become your warm-up."

BACKED UP? UNDERSTANDING HEALTHY DIGESTION

Have you ever eaten something really healthy that's not a usual part of your diet, only to find yourself rushing to the toilet a few hours later? Well, that's the opposite of backed up. The best, and by far the least pain-free, way to avoid being backed up is to have a healthy digestion. What constitutes a healthy digestion then? It is one where you are having regular bowel movements (between 2-3 times a day and once every three days). Your bowel movements should be well-formed and easy to pass. If they are loose or too difficult to pass, then this is a sign that your gut is unhealthy.

Additionally, regularly having constipation and diarrhea is a sign that your digestive system is unhealthy. This is often caused by fungus or bacteria overgrowing in your gut, causing gas, bloating, and other IBS-like symptoms.

When you have healthy digestion, you'll also feel much more energized and clear-headed without needing to rely on coffee or caffeine. Why? Because digesting your food uses a lot of energy. When you have a healthy, smooth digestion, a lot of your energy is not going towards digesting your food, which means your body can direct some of that energy to other important processes and body parts, such as your brain, lungs, and heart. A big part of our digestion is spent in cleaning mode. The second part is eating mode. Therefore, when you are not eating, your body is cleaning.

Other signs you have healthy digestion include having clear skin; move over tretinoin! There's a new beauty secret sweeping the beauty aisle: eating healthily! People who eat well do tend to, on average, have juicy, plump, clear skin.

Another less obvious sign is that you have a clean tongue. A healthy tongue looks pink and is covered with small bumps, called papillae. If you have a tongue that looks slightly different from this, such as cracks or dark marks, this could be a potential sign of bad digestive health. Having clear eyes is another indication of good digestive health. You have little to no gas. People with a healthy digestive system usually only pass gas just before a bowel movement. When they do pass gas at other times, it doesn't have an aroma. Unpleasant-smelling gas is methane-based and is an indication that your digestive health is not healthy. It is typically accompanied by bloating, distension, and pain. You are emotionally and mentally stable. Not counting days when external events may cause our emotions to be unbalanced, in general, people with healthy digestive systems experience relative emotional and mental stability.

EXERCISE & DIGESTION: CAUSE AND EFFECT

Finally! We get to talk about my favorite part! Exercise. (Although my other favorite part is food because food is delicious. We'll talk about that in Chapter Three).

Before we move on to some exercise plans, let's look at the scientific side of exercise.

There is scientific evidence that supports the theory that some exercises work to aid/treat certain digestive issues, just as there is evidence that some exercises may not be suitable for certain digestive issues. For example, running can put pressure on the abdominal muscles, which, in turn, can worsen symptoms of acid reflux or ulcerative colitis. So how does this process work?

Exercise affects the balance of bacteria in the gut. When we exercise, we trigger peristalsis, which is an involuntary muscle movement in the gut. Peristalsis moves out food through the digestive tract, improving and speeding up digestion. That's why people who workout a lot eat a lot and always seem to be hungry. With the right exercise, you can assist your peristalsis. Done consistently, you too can develop a fast metabolism to rival that of Usain Bolt's, or Olympic medalist, Michael Phelps, who eats an astounding 10,000 calories a day. That's a lot of donuts! Secondly, the benefits of exercise on gut health compound the more you perform exercise on a consistent basis. Regular exercise strengthens your digestive tract so your body doesn't divert too much blood from your gut when exercising. As a result, your digestive tract is able to continue digesting even while you exercise, promoting better health and well-being.

When exercising, you have to find the perfect balance that works for you. Some people do very well with Pilates, while others find they prefer long-distance running. Our bodies are so different that the correct response when someone asks you, "How do you find the right exercise for your gut health?" is, "It's complicated". That's the answer the Canadian Society of Intestinal Research gave, and they are the experts. As a mini-expert myself (hold your applause), let me break it down in layman's terms.

Some types of exercise can negatively affect gastric disorders, whereas others alleviate gastric disorders. When you perform intensive exercise, such as sprinting (depending on your level of fitness), all the blood leaves your gut to reach the body parts that need it most: your lungs and heart. This could cause symptoms such as nausea, diarrhea, and heartburn. On the other hand, low to moderate exercises, such as yoga, Pilates, weight-lifting, walking, jogging, swimming, and dancing, allow blood to still flow to your gut, thereby allowing you to enjoy the benefits of exercise, such as reduced bloating, as well as alleviating mental conditions that may be worsening symptoms of the gastric disorder, such as stress and anxiety. Even better, exercise releases feel-good hormones which naturally decrease stress, which is great news because your body has a faster healing process when it is less stressed. Naturally, a faster healing process improves your symptoms of digestive disorders.

On the flip side, research has also shown that high-intensity, strenuous exercise can actually reduce the main symptom of GERD, i.e., acid reflux. Furthermore, regular exercise (regardless of intensity) prevents GERD symptoms from flaring up in the long term.

Ultimately, you won't know what works for you until you plunge yourself into the world of fitness. In effect, when you do a particular type of exercise, take notes of how it makes your body feel and whether it improves or worsens symptoms of your digestive disorder. Based on its effects on your body, you can then make modifications until you find an exercise and a strain level that works well for you. I'm just a mini-expert, so my job is also to recommend you to the boss-level expert. Your doctor will be able to advise you on what exercises would work best for your condition and, just as importantly, for your particular individual needs and health history.

Exercise and gut health go together, like Monica and Chandler. In fact, having a healthy gut improves your ability - and willingness - to exercise. It's basically a beneficial loop: like a married couple that works very well together. So, maybe just a bit like Monica and Chandler. Gut health benefits exercise by helping maintain a healthy weight; when you are at a healthy weight, it's easier for you to exercise and stick to your fitness goals. Keeping your immune system strong; that way, you stay healthy and don't need to take a long time off exercising to rest and recover. Preserving your joint and bone health. This enables you to exercise without bone or joint pain hindering your progress. Producing SCFAs (Short-Chain Fatty Acid). SCFAs increase your energy levels. Being energetic is a natural motivator to stick to your exercise goals. It also powers your endurance while working out, even in conditions that may not promote endurance, such as heat and humidity. Absorbing as many nutrients from your food as possible. This also gives you the energy you need to exercise regularly.

Research is beginning to show that athletic people have a different, more healthy "gut microbiota composition" than people who live a sedentary lifestyle. Research also supports the theory that people with more diverse microbiota, including people who take probiotics, show enhanced physical performance. In other words, regular exercise improves your gut health and a healthy gut improves your exercise. Everybody wins! Especially you!

LET'S MOVE IT - GOT GUTS?

Before you put on your sports bra and your sneakers, let's look at some exercises that support digestive health and how they do that. The idea is to teach you to recognize types of exercise that are good for your digestive system. Let's start with yoga.

Yoga

Let me start by confessing that I speak from experience when I say that yoga is great for moving things along. If you are familiar with yoga, then you would know that it involves a lot of poses that require you to twist your body parts into many odd-looking formations and structures. Well, it turns out that twisting your intestines in this way promotes peristalsis. And peristalsis promotes bowel movements.

Additionally, yoga targets all areas of your muscles, releasing knots, tension, stress, and all kinds of negative emotions that we store in our muscles, nerves, and joints. This leaves us feeling much lighter psychologically, which also holistically helps our physical health, including our gut health. (As we will discuss later, your gut is intrinsically linked to your brain and your emotions.) Perhaps that's why monks are always so peaceful (at least the yoga-practicing ones). Regular yoga keeps them regular! Pun intended! If you have mild or inactive Crohn's disease, then yoga is a particularly good supplementary exercise for you.

Walking

Walking is seriously one of the best exercises ever. I'm not exaggerating!

High-intensity exercises can induce an inflammatory response in our bodies. That's why if you've ever decided to take up running or weightlifting, the day after your first session, your entire body feels as though it's throbbing and humming in pain. This is an inflammatory response.

Walking is a better exercise for people who have lived a sedentary lifestyle and want to start somewhere because it is a low-intensity exercise. From there, you can slowly incorporate more intense exercises. It is also recommended for people who have any type of inflammatory bowel disease (IBD) and cannot perform strenuous exercises that will trigger their disorder. All you need to do is start with a brisk walk down your street or around your block every day, increasing your distance and your pace by just a little bit every day.

Core Exercises

Core exercises give us stronger abdominal and back muscles. These are two very important elements if you want to have the correct form and posture when doing your other exercises. In essence, core exercises are more like supplementary exercises to benefit your main gut health exercise. They play a similar role to yoga. However, just because they are supplementary does not mean they are not essential. If you cannot achieve correct posture with a strong back and core, you won't be able to perform regular exercises in the first place.

Like yoga, your form is very important when performing core exercises. You can actually do yoga for a core workout, which is very effective. Alternatively, you can do what I do, which is incorporate Pilates abdominal exercises into core workouts.

Pilates core exercises are incredibly good for keeping your abdominal muscles strong and your guts healthy.

Deep Breathing

Meditative exercises like yoga and tai chi incorporate elements of deep breathing to promote a meditative state. Deep breathing allows you to send deep breaths to areas in your body that are tight and need release. In general, deep breathing naturally reduces stress. It has something to do with your fight-or-flight response. When you're breathing deeply, you're telling your body that you are in no way under stress or anxiety, so it naturally lets go of any stress it was holding on to, to protect you. Without stress, you boost your immune system and lower your risk of developing health problems.

Cycling

If you value your sleep and don't like nightmares, then do not search online for pictures of professional cyclists' thighs. You're probably thinking I'm exaggerating. I thought people were exaggerating too when they told me. That is, until I looked it up. It's definitely something you remember for the rest of your life. Nonetheless, don't let these pictures put you off. There is just no way you will develop thighs that massive and veiny unless you're training at a professional level.

Cycling is a very good exercise for gut health because it promotes digestion.

EXERCISE: PRACTICAL PRACTICES

We're all so very busy nowadays. We have to go to work, find time to eat, pick up our kids from school, take care of our children (if we do have children) practice our skincare routines, go out with friends or partners, stalk our ex on social media... There's just so much we have to do. And now, we also have to exercise, apparently! As if all our responsibilities are not difficult enough, many of us are having to work much harder to survive in today's financial world. It's a lot!

Exercising is supposed to improve your health, so trying to shame or force you to exercise is not going to work. It will only make your mental health suffer. Plus, what's the point of improving your physical health if your mental health will only suffer? In case you haven't heard, we're all about our mental health too! Hotties like us are so fine, not just because we do core exercises and eat our whole grains, but because we also prioritize good mental health! Good mental health will also suffer if the exercise you're doing is too hard or demanding. You're not training for the World's Strongest Man competition, so your exercise routine does not have to reflect that. And don't even get me started on the price of gym memberships and equipment today. It's like they think we're all "mobster's wife rich"!

As a hottie, you want to know how to incorporate exercise into your daily routine. Maybe you don't feel like a hottie (yet). That's perfectly natural. It just means you're a hottie-in-training. Sure, once you get that dream body, you'll be out there flaunting your stuff, but for now, maybe you just don't want anyone to see you exercising. Again, that's normal and nothing to be ashamed of. Maybe you're even low on funds, like many of us, and don't have much space to exercise. That's why this segment is full of tips to help you exercise while taking into consideration everything we've just talked about.

Here's how hotties and hotties-in-training manage to exercise. They do quick sets. Who the hell has time to exercise for two hours a day? Just 10 minutes at a time throughout your day can help you get enough exercise to keep you healthy and looking juicy. Additionally, you don't need a 200lb weight set in your home to see improvement. Bodyweight exercises are a great form of strength and muscle training. Just look at the body of any gymnast. Plus, we've already discussed the benefits of walking. A 15-minute walk post-lunch will boost your energy for the rest of the day and stop you from getting sleepy.

Do squats during meetings. Since most of us work in front of computers and phones, this enables us to multitask by exercising at work. For example, you finally booked a meeting with a very important prospective client. You want to show your client why your company is the company to take them to the next level. This is a multimillion-dollar contract, and you can't afford to blow it. So how do you bag this contract? Obviously, you do squats during the meeting. It's called multitasking, girl!

If you spend your time at work sitting, try to stand for a few hours because science has found that it is very detrimental to our health. That's why down-to-earth office spaces sometimes have chair replacements, such as treadmills, or exercise balls, to enable workers to engage and strengthen their core as well as keep their cardio up, instead of just sitting all day!

Take advantage if you work from home. Many of us are working from home these days. It's a great blessing because you can find plenty of ways to exercise at home. Want to take a quick 10 minute break from work? Do a few lunges from one end of your room to another. Enjoy a quick 10-minute yoga video workout or core exercise video. Walk to your nearby supermarket to buy some fresh berries, spinach, and yogurt to make a healthy smoothie... the possibilities are endless when you work from home!

Plan! Schedule! Calendarize! Scheduling your workout sometimes motivates us to actually workout because some of us just have a brain that likes schedules. It also gives much-needed structure for people who were teacher's pets and raised their hands to remind the teacher that she gave us homework.

If you're not a person who does really well with schedules, it can still help to plan, schedule and calendarize because it reduces the stress of making constant decisions, which, in turn, makes your workout seem less like a chore.

Boil an egg. Start small and then build up your endurance in small increments. If you tell yourself you're going to do 30 minutes of core exercise today, we both know you're not going to do it. But if you tell yourself you're going to do two minutes of core exercises today, you kind of actually just feel bad if you don't do it. It's like setting a goal to boil an egg. It's so little, you actually feel bad if you don't accomplish it. The next day, you can then decide to boil two eggs and do 3 minutes of core exercises. You get the point!

Be like a hippie. Go with the flow, man! If you scheduled a 10-minute squat session today, but don't really feel like it, then do something you feel like. Maybe it's pushups, or that plank challenge you were previously avoiding. Going with the flow and exercising is better than forcibly sticking to your schedule and not exercising.

Try different workouts. To find exercises that work for you, you have to try different ones. Don't just stick to the same boring three exercises over and over again. Doing so won't challenge your muscles, your heart, your core, etc, anyway? Even some of the world's fittest people constantly try new exercises, because you never know when you will find another great one to add to your roster.

Use what you have. Sometimes you don't need sophisticated exercise equipment. A 12-pack of water bottles carried up and down the stairs is far more difficult than you'll ever imagine. A bottle filled with rocks will give you Michelle Obama arms. Likewise, you can do things like tricep dips on the edge of your bed frame, and burpees need no equipment and very little space. Once again, the possibilities are endless.

To make your workouts much more pleasant, make sure you also do the following: Drink plenty of water, listen to workout, high RPM music. Workout with your children, partner, or friends to make it fun and motivate you. Do plenty of exercises that you like and that challenge you. Take plenty of breaks to let your body rest and your muscles recuperate. Invest in a properly-fitted sports bra, sports trainers, and exercise mat. These are just a few tips to get you in the right headspace. Incorporate whatever it is that motivates you. That way you look forward to your workouts.

EXERCISES FOR BETTER GUT HEALTH

Now that you know how to incorporate exercise into your daily life, it's time to learn what exercises you should do. Below are a variety of exercises to get you sweating and start *moving things along*. Practice these exercises, performing them at your own pace. The key is to learn the proper form so that they are safe and effective. Once you've nailed down how to do them, you will be ready to move on to the practical exercise plans that I have created just for you.

Warm-Up And Cool-Down Exercises

Cat-Cow

Focus: Stretching and lengthening of the back and neck while bringing flexibility to the spine.

1. Start in a tabletop position with your knees hip-width apart and your hands shoulder-width apart.
2. Inhale as you curve your back, drop your stomach down, tilt your pelvis up (like a cow), and look up.
3. Then slowly exhale as you arch your back and tilt your pelvis and head down (like a cat).

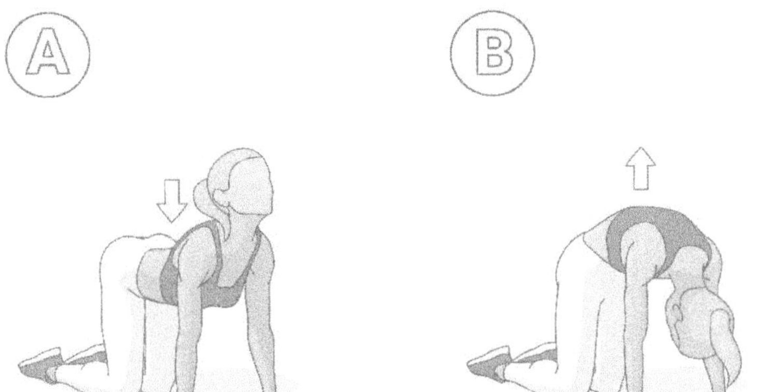

Burpees

Focus: Warms up the entire body by increasing heart rate and blood flow, preparing you for further activity while building endurance.

1. Start in a standing position with your feet hip-width apart.
2. While keeping your back straight, place your hands on the floor in front of your feet.
3. Place all your body weight on your hands, then jump your feet back to rest into a plank position on your hands.
4. Then jump back in so your feet are back in their starting position. Stand up and jump with your hands above your head.

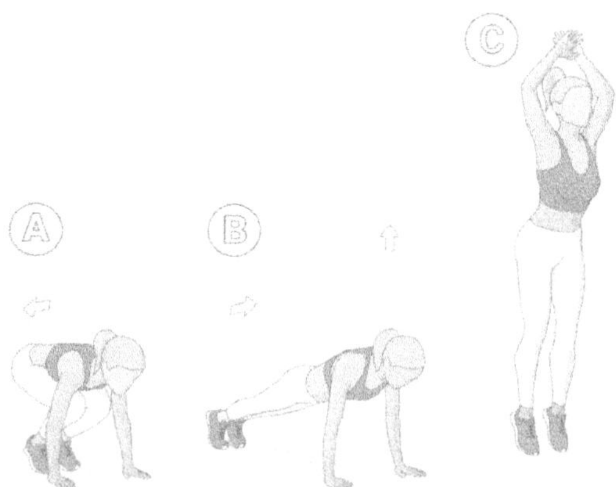

Jumping Jacks

Focus: Increases heart rate while working all major muscles in the lower body.

1. Begin by standing upright with your feet together and arms at your sides.
2. Quickly jump up while simultaneously spreading your legs to a shoulder-width distance and raising your arms over your head.
3. Jump your feet back in together and bring your arms back down to your side.

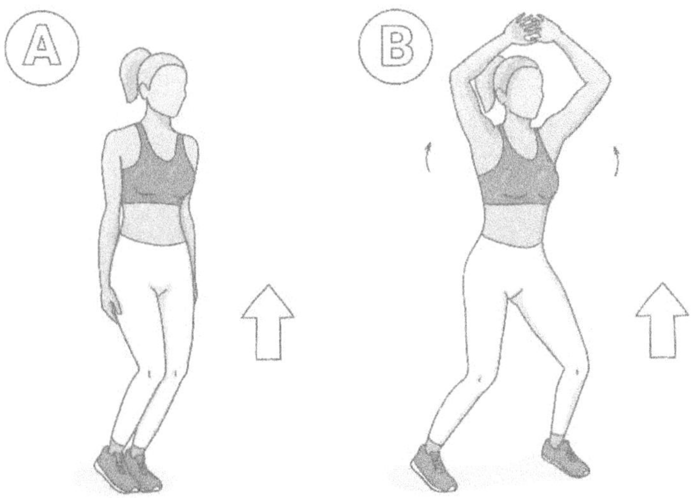

Mountain Climbers

Focus: Builds core strength while warming up all major muscle groups.

1. Start in a high plank position with your hands shoulder-width apart and your shoulders inline with your wrists.
2. Draw one knee toward your chest while keeping your foot on the ground. Quickly switch legs by jumping and bringing the opposite knee towards your chest while extending the first leg back.
3. Continue to alternate legs as quickly as possible while maintaining proper form and keeping your core engaged.

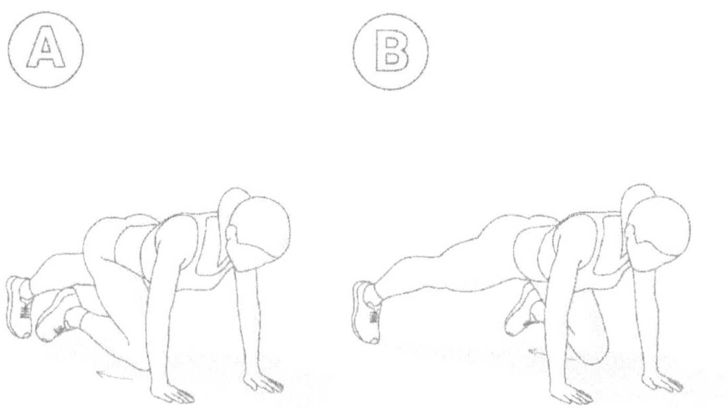

High Knees

Focus: Builds endurance and activates abdominals and major lower body muscle groups.

1. Stand up straight with your feet hip-width apart and your arms hanging down by your side.
2. Start jogging in place, lifting your knees up towards your hips as high as you can while keeping your core engaged. As you lift each knee up, alternate your feet so that your right knee is up when your left foot is down, and vice versa.

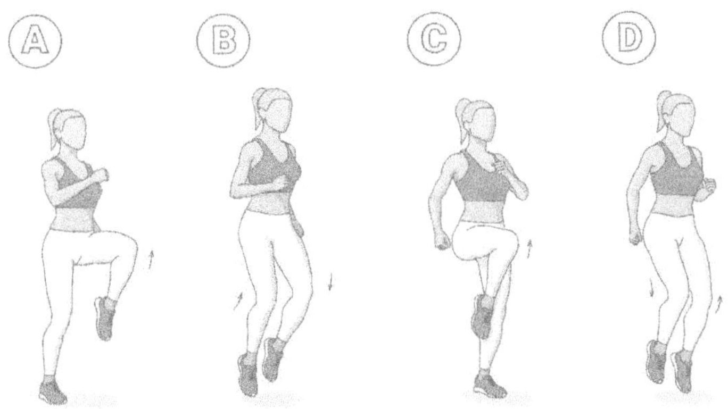

Inchworm

Focus: Full body warmup activates most major muscle groups in both the upper and lower body and strengthens core muscles.

1. Standing tall with your feet hip-width apart, reach down and place your hands on the floor in front of your feet.
2. Walk your hands forward until you are in a high plank position. Remember to keep your core engaged.
3. Slowly start to walk your hands back until they are in front of your feet. Come back up to a standing position.

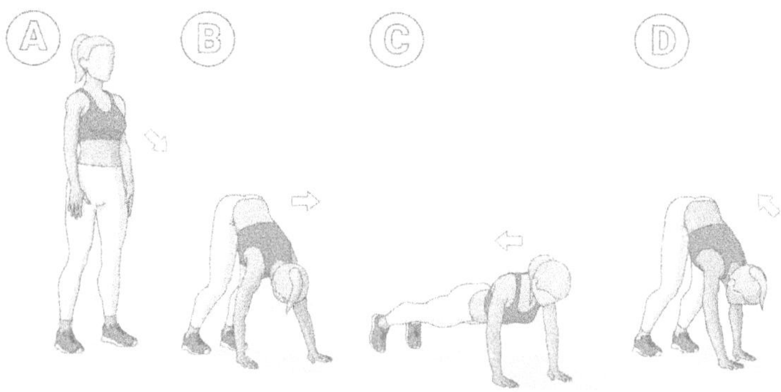

Run on The Spot

Focus: Elevates heart rate and activates major muscle groups in the lower body.

1. Start with your feet hip-width apart and a slight bend in the knees.
2. Raise one knee up, lifting the foot slightly off the ground, and quickly switch legs while swinging the arms.
3. Repeat continuously until the exercise is complete.

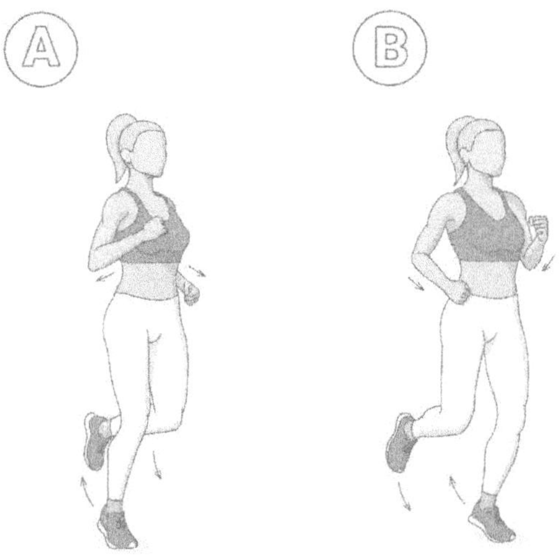

Downward Dog

Focus: Stretches the hamstrings, calves, and Achilles tendons.

1. Position yourself in a high plank, with your fingers spread on the floor.
2. Shift your hips and buttocks upwards in the air in an inverted V shape.
3. Press your weight into your fingers and palms, then press your heels into the ground. You will feel a deep stretch in your calf. The closer your calves move to the ground, the deeper you will feel the stretch in both calves. Bend your knees slightly, but continue to press your heels towards the ground.

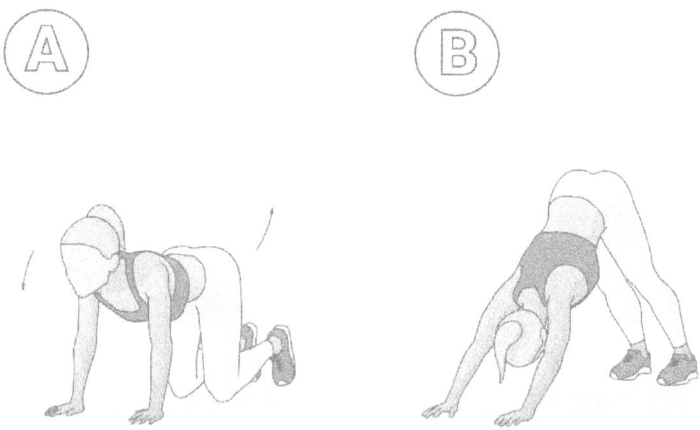

Quadricep Stretch

Focus: Lengthens and stretches the quadricep muscle in the front of the leg.

1. Stand tall and hold on to something for balance.
2. Bend your knee and grasp your ankle with one hand.
3. Keep your knees in line and your back up straight.

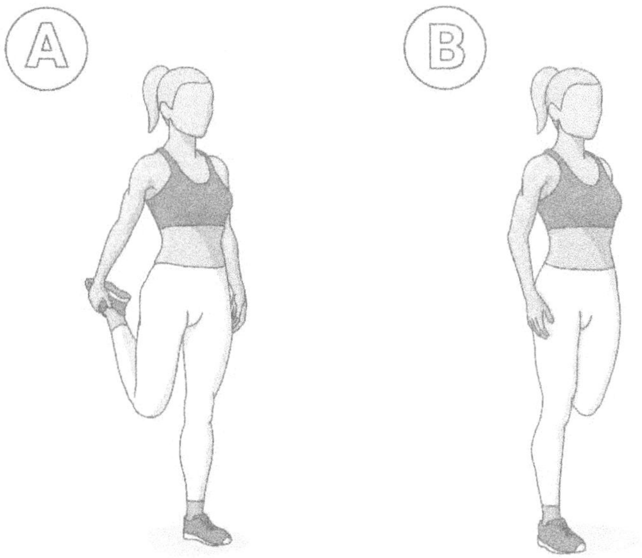

Seated Forward Bend

Focus: Stretches hamstrings, lengthening the spine and relaxing the central nervous system.

1. Start in the seated position on a solid surface with your feet both in front of you and your legs straight.
2. Inhale as you lift both of your arms above your head. Exhale and fold forward from your waist, reaching for your toes. Do not try to force yourself down. Simply allow your body to reach as far as it can go.

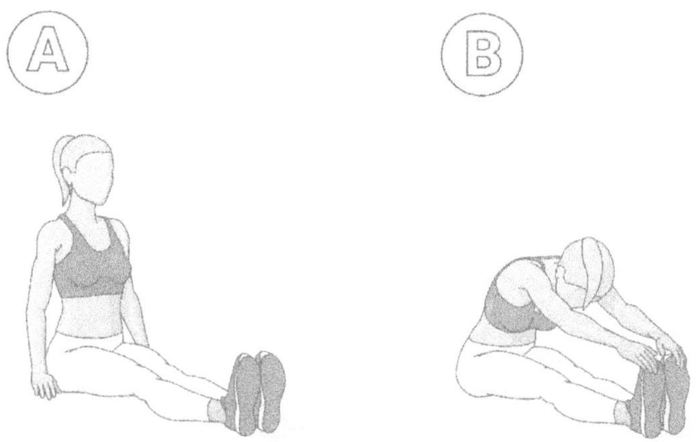

Upward-Facing Dog

Focus: Stretches pectorals and abdominal muscles. Strengthens shoulders, arms, and back muscles.

1. Ly flat on your stomach and place your hands palms down beside your waist.
2. Draw your chest up and forward while keeping your shoulders pushed back and down.

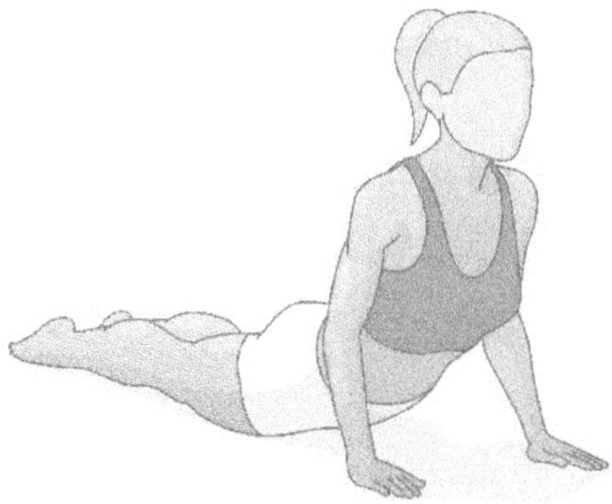

Lower Body Exercises

Squats

Focus: Strengthens gluteus maximus, quadriceps, hamstrings, calves, and core muscles.

1. Start in a standing position with your feet slightly wider than shoulder-width apart and your toes slightly pointed outwards.
2. Slowly squat down like you are going to sit in a chair, with only a slight lean forward with the upper body.
3. Keep your body weight on to your heels and push your knees outward while returning to the standing position.

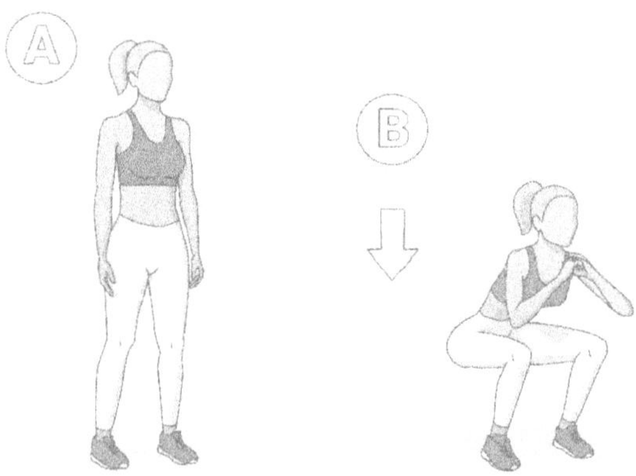

Jump Squats

Focus: Strengthens gluteus maximus, quadriceps, hamstrings, calves, and core muscles and improves cardiovascular fitness.

1. Start in a standing position with your feet slightly wider than shoulder-width apart and your toes slightly pointed outwards.
2. Squat down like you are going to sit in a chair, with only a slight lean forward with the upper body.
3. Keep your body weight on to your heels and push your knees outward.
4. Jump up with your arms swinging backward so that your feet come off the floor. Land back into a squat position and repeat.

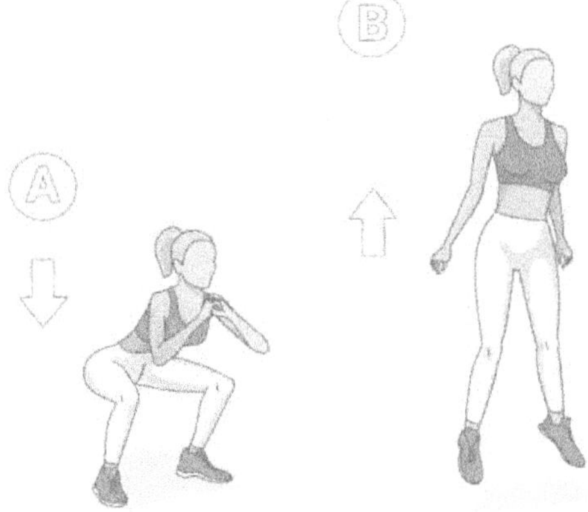

Glute Bridges

Focus: Strengthens gluteus maximus and core muscles. Improves posture and balance, as well as reduces back pain.

1. Start by lying on your back with your knees bent and your feet flat on the floor, hip-width apart.
2. Push your heels into the floor and raise your hips up as high as you can, squeezing your glute muscles.
3. Slowly return hips back to the floor and repeat.

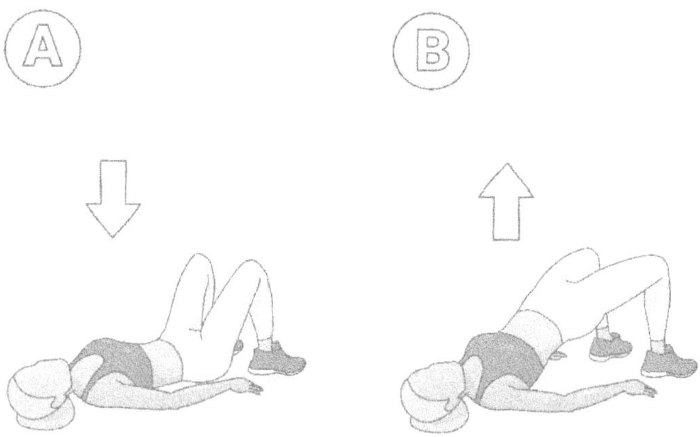

Lunges to Knee Drive

Focus: Strengthens gluteus maximus and quadriceps. Improves balance and cardiovascular fitness.

1. Start in a lunge position with your front knee in line with your heel and your back knee in line with your hip.
2. Keeping your weight on the front leg, slightly lean forward.
3. Quickly push off of your front leg and drive the opposite knee forward and up.
4. Return to the starting lunge position and repeat.

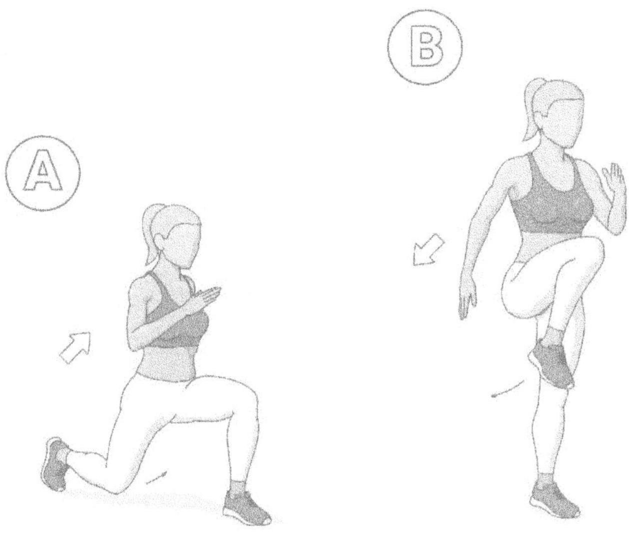

Upper Body Exercises

Push-ups

Focus: Strengthens pectorals, serratus anterior, rotator cuffs, and core.

1. Start in the high plank position, keeping your neck straight and your gaze down.
2. With your arms slightly wider than shoulder-width apart, slowly lower your body close to the floor, then push back up to the starting position.
3. Remember to keep your core muscles engaged throughout this exercise.

Tip: To modify this exercise, bend your knees and rest them on the floor.

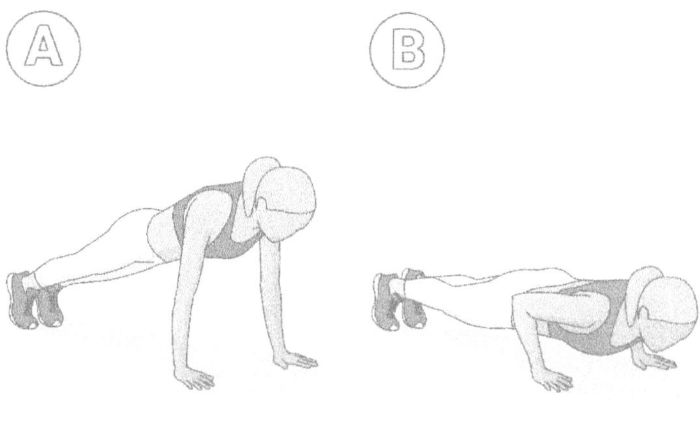

Triceps Dips

Focus: Strengthens pectoral muscles, triceps, and shoulders while activating the core muscles.

1. Begin seated on top of a solid, unmoving base, such as a bed frame or chair.
2. Place your palms on the edge of the frame. Your elbows will go back, while your forearms and palms will stay aligned with your shoulders.
3. Straighten your legs out in front of you so that your heels are resting on the ground.
4. Begin to dip down, then press back up, letting your triceps lift your weight.

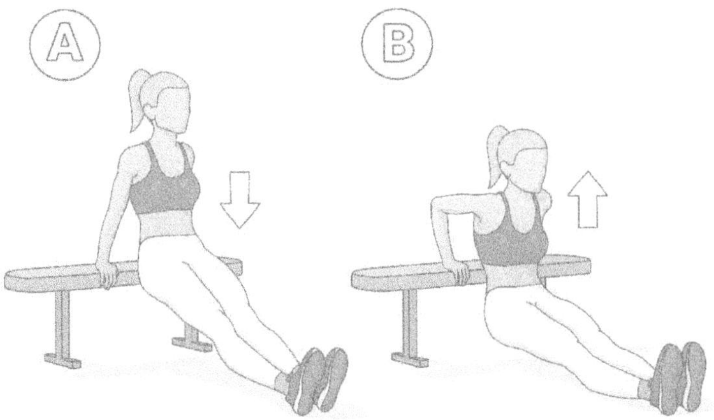

Plank Walk

Focus: Strengthens shoulders, pectorals, triceps, and core.

1. Start in a plank position on your elbows and toes.
2. Raise one arm and push the floor with the palm of your hand, straightening your arm, then place the other hand on the floor so they align with each other.
3. Lower back down to the starting position and repeat by alternating sides.

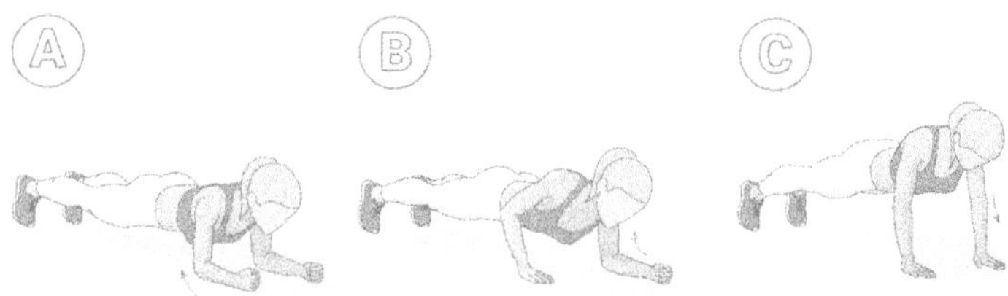

Plank Tap

Focus: Strengthens shoulders, arms, and core muscles.

1. Begin in a high plank position, resting on your palms.
2. Keep your body still and your back straight as you lift your right palm off the ground and gently tap your left shoulder. Return your right palm to the ground and repeat with your left palm, tapping your right shoulder gently. Continue alternating.

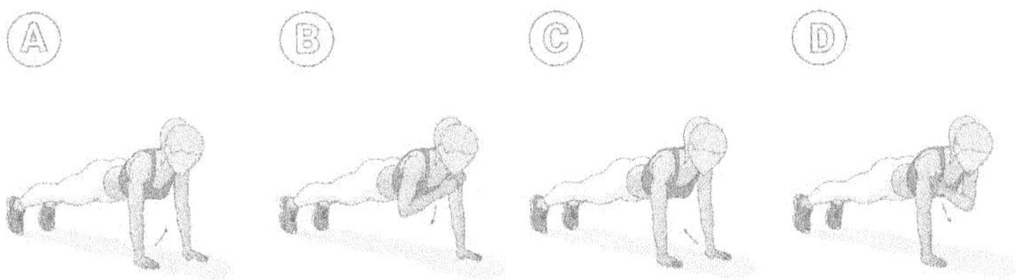

Core Exercises

Seated Crunches

Focus: Strengthens and stabilizes the lower back and abdominal muscles. Improves posture and balance.

1. Sit on the floor with your legs straight out in front. Keep your hands on the ground beside you, just behind your hips.
2. With your weight resting on your hands, raise your legs, bending your knees in towards your stomach and pushing your upper body towards your bent knees.
3. Push your legs and upper body back to their original positions, then repeat.

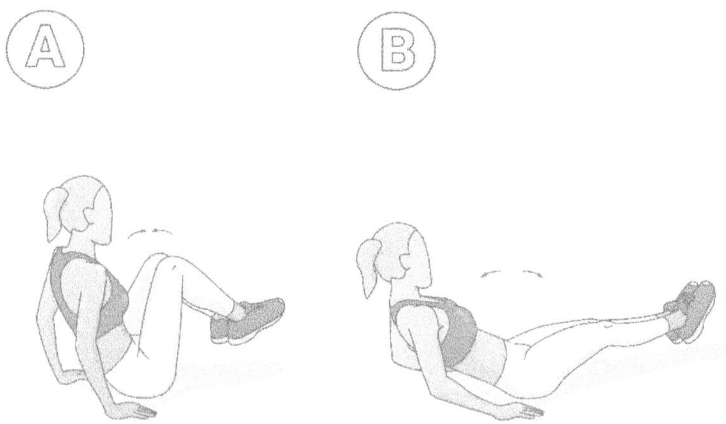

Dead Bug

Focus: Strengthens and stabilizes core, spine, and back muscles.

1. Lying on your back, raise your feet off the ground and bring your knees upwards until your calves are horizontal to the ground. Stretch your arms up to the sky vertically.
2. Tilt your pelvis towards the ground so that your lower back is flat on the floor.
3. Lower the left leg down until it is just above the ground. At the same time, move your right arm in the opposite direction, bringing it downwards, horizontally, until it is just above the ground.
4. Bring your left leg and right arm back to position and repeat with your right leg and left arm. Continue alternating.

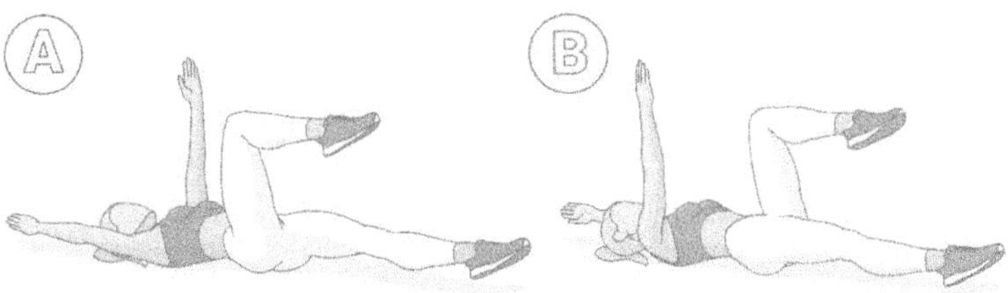

Russian Twist

Focus: Strengthens obliques and abdominal muscles.

1. Start by sitting on the floor with your feet touching the ground. Keeping your back flat, slightly lean back and clasp your hands together in front of your chest.
2. Engage your abdominal muscles and twist your torso to the left side, bringing your clasped hands to the left side of your body.
3. Hold the twist for one second, then twist back to the center and then to the right side. Continue repeating the movement.

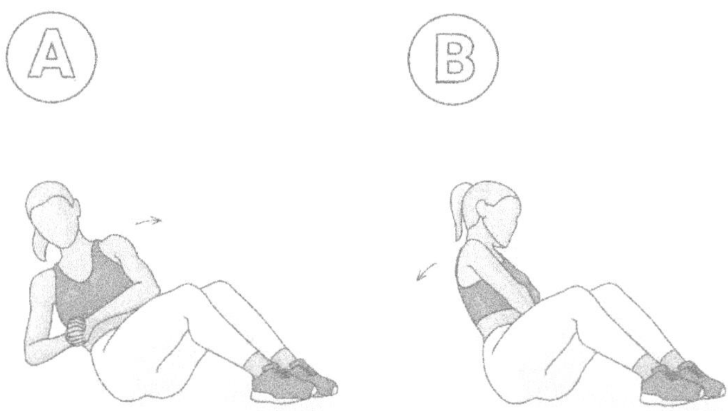

Plank

Focus: Strengthens the TVA (transversus abdominus), rectus abdominus and oblique muscles.

1. Place both elbows on the ground in line with your shoulders. Slide your legs back and lift your knees so you are resting on your elbows and toes.
2. Keep your back straight (so a tea tray set on it will not fall over), then activate your core muscles by breathing in and pulling in your core muscles with your breath.

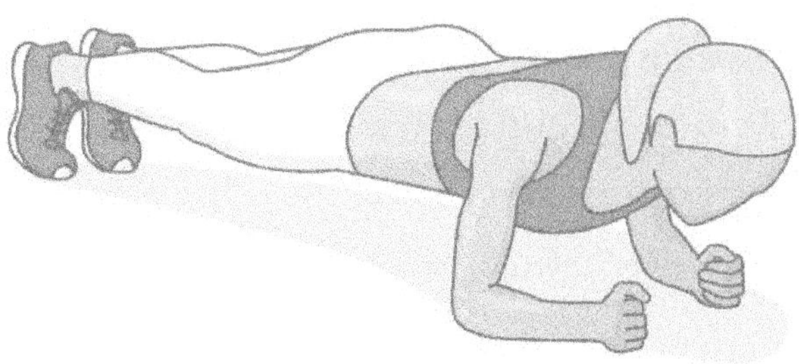

Birddog

Focus: Strengthens core muscles while activating most major muscle groups. Improves stability and relieves low back pain.

1. Start on your hands and knees in a tabletop position. Your hands should be directly under your shoulders, and your knees directly under your hips.
2. Engage your core and keep your spine in a neutral position.
3. Extend your left leg behind you, keeping it straight and reaching it out as far as you comfortably can. At the same time, raise your right arm out in front of you, keeping it straight.
4. Hold this position for two seconds, then slowly lower your arm and leg back down to the starting position. Repeat on the other side, then continue alternating sides.

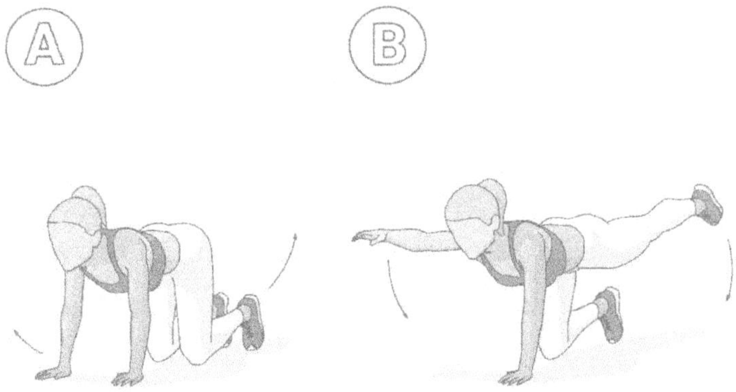

EXERCISE PLAN: 10, 30, 60

Now that you have practiced how to perform each exercise, this is where we put it all together. Here is where you start your journey into becoming a gut-healthy hottie with these three beginner-friendly workouts. These three workouts last for 10 minutes, 30 minutes, and 60 minutes. Being beginner-friendly, they are easy to follow, require minimal space, and don't need any fancy/complicated exercise equipment. Let's get started!

10-Minute Exercise Plan

Warmup (1 Minute): Cat-Cow (30 seconds), jumping jacks (30 seconds).

Complete each circuit by performing each exercise and rest period for 20 seconds. Repeat each circuit twice.

Circuit 1 (4 Minutes): Burpee, plank, rest, squats, plank, rest.

Circuit 2 (4 Minutes): Mountain climbers, seated crunches, rest, high knees, plank walk, rest.

Cooldown (1 Minute): Seated forward bend (30 seconds), downward dog (30 seconds).

30-Minute Exercise Plan

Warmup (3 min): Cat-Cow (30 seconds), downward dog (30 seconds), jumping jacks (60 seconds), burpees (60 seconds).

Complete each circuit by performing each exercise and rest period for 40 seconds each. Repeat each circuit three times.

Circuit 1 (8 Minutes): High knees, push-ups, plank walk, rest.

Circuit 2 (8 Minutes): Mountain climbers, lunges to knee drive (20 seconds each leg), squats, rest.

Circuit 3 (8 Minutes): Dead bug, Russian twist, seated crunch, rest.

Cool down (3 min): Upward facing dog (30 seconds), downward facing dog (30 seconds), seated forward bend (60 seconds), quadriceps stretch (30 seconds on each side).

60-Minute Exercise Plan

Warmup (4 minutes): Perform each warmup exercise for 60 seconds; end the warmup with a 60-second rest. Inchworm, burpees, jumping jacks.

Complete each circuit by performing each exercise for 50 seconds, followed by 10 seconds of rest. Rest for 1 minute before repeating the circuit. Repeat each circuit 3 times.

Circuit 1 Lower Body (18 Minutes): Jump squats, lunges with knee drive, glute bridges, mountain climbers, high knees. Rest for 1 minute.

Circuit 2 Upper Body (18 Minutes): Plank walk, push-ups, triceps dips, inchworm, plank taps. Rest for 1 minute.

Circuit 3 Core (18 Minutes): Dead bug, Russian twist, seated crunch, Birddog, plank.

Cooldown (2 minutes): Upward dog (30 seconds), downward dog (30 seconds), quadricep stretch (30 seconds each side).

As we've seen in this chapter, exercise is crucial for gut health. However, it goes hand-in-hand with diet. As you begin to incorporate exercise into your life, the next stage in your hottie transformation (or, as I like to classily call it, your hottie-sformation) is to change your diet. In the next chapter, I have curated for you a 30-day meal plan guaranteed to improve digestion and get rid of bloating for a flatter tummy. Let's go!

3

MADE IN THE KITCHEN: 30-DAY FLAT TUMMY MEAL PLAN

> *"Abs are made in the kitchen."*
>
> — ANONYMOUS

Putting aside the utmost and utter importance of a flat tummy for one second (Yes, I know! Blasphemy!), it's always a good idea to eat nutritiously. Good nutrition is pivotal to our gut health and, as we will see in later chapters, our overall health.

OK, now that that's done, let me climb off my soapbox so we can proceed. As the saying goes: "Abs are made in the kitchen!"

DIETING FOR GUT HEALTH

I threw in this section to see if you've been paying attention so far! If you thought to yourself, "eat probiotics and whole wheats for gut health," then you passed the test. If not, you can go back to the section in Chapter One, Gut Bacteria: Helpful vs. Harmful, to reacquaint yourself with tips on how to diet for gut health.

Another wonderful tip for dieting to improve your gut health is practicing mindful eating. I had a friend a few years ago whom I would often meet for lunch and a coffee. I'm not exaggerating when I share with you that she took 35 minutes to chew a simple sandwich. It was frustrating to watch. Now that I look back, I realize that Sarah was practicing mindful eating. This involves chewing your food well, so that you don't overload the rest of your digestive process, including your stomach and intestines. People often forget that chewing is the first part of the digestive process called mastication. Its purpose is to break down your food so that it's easier to digest in your stomach and intestines. People who don't chew their food properly, are left with bloating, gas, and other digestive symptoms. When in doubt, chew like a cow!

Avoid trigger foods. Trigger foods are foods that create an imbalance in your gut microbiota. Sugar is the worst of them all. It is like feeding the pathogenic bacteria in your gut super steroid protein shakes. Other forms of pathogenic super steroid protein shakes are:

- Processed foods
- Artificial sweeteners
- Gluten-containing grains (if you're gluten-sensitive)
- Dairy products (apart from yogurt and kefir)
- Foods high in saturated fats and trans fat, which only increase inflammation caused by gastric disorders

Now, we just need a scientist to make sugar less addictive than cocaine (seriously, look it up), then we can all finally kick our cravings!

Eat foods high in healthy fats, such as omega-3 and monounsaturated fats (such as olive oil and flax seeds) to reduce inflammation in your digestive system.

Avoid foods that cause heartburn. Heartburn allows food to sit for longer in your stomach, leading to a host of digestive issues. Foods that often cause heartburn include:

- Fried food
- Fast food
- Processed food
- Citrus fruits
- Peppermint
- Chili powder
- White, black, and cayenne pepper
- Chocolate
- Fatty meats, e.g., bacon
- Cheese
- Tomato-based sauces
- Chocolate
- Carbonated beverages

You can still eat these foods from time to time, but moderation is key. You may also want to avoid eating them before bedtime because lying down after eating these foods will lead to severe heartburn.

When in doubt, chew like a cow! However, this time it just means eating a wide diversity of plants. Here is the advice that dietician Dr. Heather Finley gave: Aim to eat 30 different plants per week (from fruits, vegetables, nuts, seeds, legumes, and herbs) - or as many varieties as you possibly can. It's a good thing my meal plan is packed with diverse plants! Cows also like to graze, meaning they eat smaller meals in greater frequency instead of larger meals a couple of times a day.

Lastly, quit late-night dinners and bedtime snacks. As your body prepares to sleep, it slows down all bodily functions, including your metabolism. This bad habit can quickly lead to weight gain and poor digestion. So put down the chocolate brownies and choose a cup of healthy ginger tea before bed!

HOW TO MANAGE COMMON DIGESTIVE DISORDERS

In Chapter One, we discussed IBS and dysbiosis. However, they are not the only common digestive issues that impact gut health and overall physical health. Those, along with other digestive disorders, can be managed with a healthy diet. Other potential problems related to digestive disorders include:

Small intestinal bacterial overgrowth (SIBO)

Our food regularly moves forward through our digestive tract. This is called motility. When an issue prevents them from moving forward, bacteria begin to colonize in the small intestine, attracted to the food. As our small intestine is not able to handle too much bacteria at once, this leads to constipation, diarrhea, or bloating.

People diagnosed with IBS are most likely to be diagnosed with SIBO. In any case, doctors still are not always exactly sure what causes SIBO. Common symptoms tend to be diarrhea, bloating, constipation, and vitamin deficiencies, in particular, vitamin B12 deficiency.

If symptoms of SIBO are not well-controlled, or if they are severe, it could lead to dehydration, rapid weight loss, low energy, and nutritional deficiencies. A person

with these symptoms is physically unable to perform exercise, leading to even lower motility.

Gastroesophageal Reflux Disease (GERD)

GERD is a disease that occurs when a person frequently has acid reflux. It begins when your stomach contents repeatedly come back up into your esophagus and food pipe. The stomach's pH is very high, which means that the acid coming back up is also very acidic. This causes the esophagus to get inflamed or irritated (a condition known as esophagitis). At any rate, some people do develop GERD without esophagitis.

Common symptoms of GERD include chest pain, acid reflux, heartburn, nausea, and pain while swallowing. Quitting smoking and making dietary changes are common ways in which GERD is treated. Over-the-counter medications are also effective. With the right treatment, a person with GERD should have no problem with physical exercise. However, if the condition becomes severe, including symptoms such as, more frequent acid reflux, unexplained weight loss, difficulty swallowing, vomiting, and common symptoms worsening, cease exercising and call your doctor.

Gallstones

The gallbladder is a very important part of digestion. It produces bile which we use to digest and absorb fat, especially when you give in to your inner food demon and order that bacon cheeseburger I told you not to. Gallstones sometimes form in the gallbladder, however, and, unfortunately, it's possible to have gallstones and not be aware of it because our bodies show no symptoms. Where your body shows symptoms is if your gallstones form in an opening in your gallbladder, blocking the ducts connecting your gallbladder to your intestines. If this happens, you will notice symptoms, such as vomiting, jaundice (which will cause you to look like a character on The Simpsons), nausea, high temperature, sweating, and consistent pain just below the ribs on the right side of the body.

If you notice these symptoms 2-3 times a week, consistently, speak with your doctor. Conversely, if you notice the following symptoms, contact your doctor immediately: jaundice, chills/a high temperature, and pain in the abdomen that lasts for more than 8 hours.

Celiac Disease

Celiac disease is classified as an autoimmune condition. People with coeliac disease have an immune system that reacts negatively towards gluten. Celiac disease can be a very dangerous condition because repeated exposure will eventually damage the small intestine. Once the small intestine is damaged, it usually causes problems absorbing nutrients and minerals from food.

Symptoms of celiac disease include weight loss, fatigue/anemia, depression, anxiety, abdominal pain, chronic diarrhea or constipation, nausea and vomiting, bloating and gas, pale stool with a very bad smell, fatty stool that floats and nerve damage, causing tingling in the legs and feet.

The symptoms of celiac disease are quite severe, so much so that they would prevent you from exercising even mildly. If you notice these symptoms, book an appointment with your doctor to review your diet plan. You can lead a healthy, fulfilling life full of physical activity even with this condition. All you need to do is avoid gluten. For white bread lovers, this may sound like punishment for previous sins, but that is the price you pay for a healthy life with celiac disease.

The treatment for celiac disease is simple: avoid gluten forever. Foods that contain gluten include barley, bulgur, rye, durum, farina, semolina, graham flour, malt, wheat, spelt (a form of wheat), and triticale (a hybrid of wheat and rye).

The following foods, medication, and non-food products sometimes contain gluten, so be alert when using them. Modified food starch, food preservatives, food stabilizers, some toothpaste and mouthwash, prescription and over-the-counter medications, herbal and nutritional supplements, vitamin and mineral supplements, lipstick products, envelope and stamp glue, and play dough.

Why do so many things contain gluten? It's like the whole world woke up and thought: "You know what we should do for jokes? Put gluten in everything, even though it is potentially fatal to people with celiac disease!" I stand in solidarity with my celiac disease sisters! Together, we can defeat this oppression!

Crohn's disease

Crohn's disease is one of a few types of inflammatory bowel disease (IBD). People with Crohn's disease suffer from chronic inflammation of the GI tract. You would know you have Crohn's disease if you have the following symptoms: blood in your stool, unexplained weight loss, fatigue, abdominal pain, chronic diarrhea, chest pains, shortness of breath, blocked bowel, rectal bleeding, bone fracture, cold hands and feet, and dizziness. Crohn's disease can be genetic, and it can be caused by environmental factors. It may also be caused by an autoimmune reaction to some bacteria in the digestive tract.

If you have Crohn's disease, medicines may work to reduce inflammation. In more severe cases, where drugs don't work, you may need what is called "bowel rest," which gives your intestines a chance to heal. Alternatively, some people need surgery as a treatment for Crohn's disease.

Ulcerative colitis (UC)

Ulcerative colitis is another type of inflammatory bowel disease (IBD). It causes the large intestine and the rectum to become inflamed. Not only that, but this inflammation will spread to other areas of the intestines after some time. Typical symptoms of UC include consistent, long-term diarrhea, abdominal pain, tiredness, and unexplained weight loss.

Ulcerative colitis is typically caused by an autoimmune response. Like Crohn's disease and other types of IBD, it can also be caused by environmental factors and genetics. Since symptoms of UC are not debilitating, they should not affect regular fitness even without treatment. However, if you experience severe or recurring flare-ups of the above symptoms, contact your doctor.

YOUR 30-DAY MEAL PLAN FOR A FLATTER TUMMY

We made it! We finally get to the really good part: the food part! I have curated this meal plan based on all the scientific information in this book, so you are guaranteed you are eating the best meals for your gut microbiome. I put together recipes that will help you reduce bloating, fight inflammation, lose weight (in a safe, gradual fashion), give you more energy, and improve your mood.

If you don't have plenty of practice cooking, there's no need to worry. The meals in your meal plan are easy to prepare, with simple cooking styles and affordable and easily accessible ingredients. You don't need any training or fancy equipment to prepare your meals, and the lunch options can be easily prepared as a packed lunch.

Before we begin, do always remember to practice safe nutrition and dieting. Check with your primary physician or a professional before making any major changes to your nutrition (especially if you have food allergies, are on medication, or are on a special diet). Below are all the gut-healthy recipes at your disposal. Once you make your way through the recipes, you will find your meal plan awaits you!

With that being said, let's begin!

Breakfast Recipes

Overnight oats with berries and chia seeds

Servings: 1

Ingredients

- ½ cup uncooked oats
- ½ cup almond milk
- ½ cup plain non-fat Greek yogurt
- 1 tablespoon spoon chia seeds
- ½ teaspoon cinnamon
- 1 cup fresh mixed berries

Directions

Add oats to your container of choice and pour in the milk. Layer chia seeds, Greek yogurt, and berries on top. Refrigerate overnight.

Nutritional Information

Calories: 378 kcal, Fat: 14g, Carbs: 50g, Sugars: 18g, Protein: 17g, Fiber: 8g, Sodium: 120mg

Avocado toast with poached eggs

Servings: 1

Ingredients

- 2 slices whole grain bread
- 2 eggs
- ½ avocado
- salt and pepper, to taste
- Herbs, to season
- Heirloom tomatoes, quartered (optional)

Directions

Boil water in a pot, using enough water to cover your eggs as they poach.

Turn off the heat once the water boils. Carefully crack two eggs into the pot of water. Cover the pot for 4-5 minutes, depending on whether you want soft-boiled or hard-boiled eggs. As the eggs cook, toast the bread and lay them flat on a plate. Smash the avocado and layer on each piece of toast. Lift the eggs out of the pot of hot water using a slotted cooking spoon, then place the eggs onto the avocado toast. Season with salt, pepper, and herbs. Serve with heirloom tomatoes, if desired.

Nutritional Information

Calories: 393 kcal, Fat: 17g, Carbs: 30g, Sugars:5g, Protein: 20g, Fiber: 8g, Sodium: 400mg

Sweet potato pancakes

Servings: 1

Ingredients

- 1 medium peeled sweet potato, cooked and cooled
- 2 large eggs
- Sprinkle of cinnamon
- Sprinkle of nutmeg
- 1 tbsp tablespoon of oil

- ½ cup non-fat Greek Yogurt (optional for the topping)
- 1 teaspoon maple syrup/honey

Directions

In a medium bowl, mash sweet potato, then whisk in eggs and nutmeg.

Heat a griddle pan on medium-high with olive oil. Cook on each side for 3-5 minutes. To serve with topping, mix yogurt with maple syrup/honey and a sprinkle of cinnamon. Spoon next to pancakes.

Nutritional Information

Calories: 350 kcal, Fat: 13g, Carbs: 34g, Sugars: 17g, Protein: 26g, Fiber: 4g, Sodium: 230mg

Berry Kefir Smoothie

Servings: 1

Ingredients

- 1½ cups frozen blueberries
- 1 cup plain kefir
- 1 medium banana
- 2 teaspoons almond butter
- ½ teaspoon vanilla extract

- 1 teaspoon chia seeds
- Sprinkle of cinnamon

Directions

Combine blueberries, kefir, banana, chia seeds, almond butter, and vanilla in a blender. Blend until smooth. Sprinkle cinnamon and enjoy.

Nutritional Information

Calories: 350 kcal, Fat: 7g, Carbs: 60g, Sugars: 40g, Protein: 17g, Fiber: 10g, Sodium: 25mg

Peanut butter banana cinnamon toast

Servings: 1

Ingredients

- 1 medium banana, sliced
- 2 slices whole wheat bread, toasted
- 1 tablespoon natural peanut butter (or any other nut butter)
- Sprinkle of cinnamon

Directions

Spread peanut butter on toast. Add banana slices evenly on both slices, then sprinkle with cinnamon.

Nutritional Information

Calories: 366 kcal, Fat: 10g, Carbs: 40g, Sugars: 20g, Protein: 10g, Fiber: 10g, Sodium: 120mg

Gluten-free lemon blueberry muffins

Servings: 6

Ingredients

- 1½ cups gluten-free flour blend
- ½ teaspoon salt
- 2 teaspoons baking powder
- ½ teaspoon baking soda
- 1 large lemon, zested and juiced
- 1 ½ cup blueberries
- 1 cup granulated sugar
- 1 tablespoon sugar
- 5 tablespoons vegan or oat butter
- 2 large eggs
- ⅓ cup almond milk

Directions

Preheat oven to 400°F., Line a 6-cup muffin pan with muffin liners, then set aside.

Sift the dry ingredients (except sugar) into a large bowl. Stir to combine. In another bowl, whisk milk and lemon juice. Beat eggs then add the beaten eggs to the milk and lemon mixture. Whisk until well combined. Sprinkle 1 cup of sugar onto blueberries, then mix thoroughly. Fold in the blueberries, sugar, and lemon zest into the batter.

Pour the batter evenly into the muffin pans. Bake for 25-30 minutes.

Nutritional Information

Calories: 310 kcal, Fat: 13g, Carbs: 48g, Sugars: 25g, Protein: 6g, Fiber: 5g, Sodium: 415mg

Tomato and leek frittata

Servings: 4

Ingredients

- 3 egg whites
- 2 egg yolks
- 3 teaspoons olive oil, divided
- 1⁄2 teaspoon sea salt, divided
- 1⁄2 cup chopped leek leaves
- 1⁄2 teaspoon freshly ground black pepper, divided

- 1⁄2 cup grape tomatoes
- 1 teaspoon dried herbs
- 1 teaspoon dried thyme
- 2 ounces goat cheese, crumbled

Directions

Preheat oven to 350°F., In a 10" ovenproof non-stick skillet, heat 2 teaspoons of oil over medium heat. Add leeks and cook for 5 minutes, adding ¼ teaspoon salt and ¼ teaspoon pepper. Stir in grape tomatoes. Cover and cook for another 3 minutes then transfer to a small bowl. In a medium bowl, add egg whites, thyme, herbs, and remaining salt and pepper. Whisk rapidly. Whisk in egg yolks, then continue to whisk until mixture is fluffy. Brush skillet with remaining olive oil, then add tomato mixture, eggs mixture and goat cheese. Cook over medium heat for 4 minutes then transfer to oven. Bake for 15–20 minutes or until eggs are set. You will know the eggs are set by cutting a small slit in the center of the frittata.

Nutritional Information

Calories: 300 kcal, Fat: 30g, Carbs: 4g, Sugars: 2g, Protein: 30g, Fiber: 1g, Sodium: 1000mg

Ginger and Mango Smoothie

Servings: 1

Ingredients

- 1½ cup mango, fresh or frozen
- 1 inch fresh ginger
- 2 cups unsweetened almond milk, or water
- ½ lime, juiced
- 3 tablespoons oats
- 1 tablespoon hemp seeds, optional
- 1 teaspoon cinnamon, optional

Directions

Add all the ingredients into a blender. Blend on high until smooth.

Nutritional Information

Calories: 450 kcal, Fat: 30g, Carbs: 75g, Sugars: 40g, Protein: 37g, Fiber: 20g, Sodium: 50mg

Overnight oats with bananas, almonds, and almond butter

Servings: 1

Ingredients

- 2 teaspoons almond butter
- 1 medium banana, sliced
- ½ cup soya milk
- Handful of almonds, crushed
- 1 tablespoon chia seeds
- ½ cups, oats
- Sprinkle of cinnamon

Directions

Layer almond butter at the bottom of a mason jar. Layer bananas on top of the almond butter. In a small bowl, add milk, oats, chia seeds and cinnamon. Stir to mix well. Layer oat milk mixture on top of bananas. Refrigerate overnight, then serve.

Nutritional Information

Calories: 499 kcal, Fat: 20g, Carbs: 70g, Sugars: 28g, Protein: 13g, Fiber: 10g, Sodium: 220mg

Strawberry smoothie with chia seeds and Greek yogurt

Servings: 1

Ingredients

- 2 cups almond milk (or a non-dairy alternative of your choice)
- 1 cup Greek Yogurt
- 1 cup frozen strawberries
- ½ orange, peeled, optional
- ¼ cup oats, optional
- 2 tablespoons chia seeds
- 1 tablespoon honey, optional
- ½ teaspoon vanilla extract, optional

Directions

Blend all the ingredients together in a blender, until smooth. Serve immediately.

Nutritional Information

Calories: 400 kcal, Fat: 25g, Carbs: 35g, Sugars: 20g, Protein: 15g, Fiber: 10g, Sodium: 10mg

Lunch Recipes

Thai carrot soup

Servings: 6

Ingredients

- 1 small-medium onion, chopped
- 1 celery stalk, chopped
- 1 lb carrot, chopped into 1-inch pieces
- 2 tablespoons peanut butter
- 1 inch fresh ginger piece, peeled and thinly sliced
- 1 medium chili pepper, sliced, or 1 teaspoon red pepper flakes
- 1 garlic clove, thinly chopped
- 1 teaspoon olive oil
- 2 tablespoons soy sauce
- 1 teaspoon sesame oil
- 1½ cup vegetable broth
- 1 can coconut milk, unsweetened
- Fresh cilantro leaves to decorate, chopped, optional

Directions

In a large pot, sauté onions, garlic and celery in olive and garlic oil. Sauté over low-medium heat, stirring constantly to prevent the vegetables from burning. Add ginger, carrots, red pepper flakes and vegetable broth. Cover the pot, then simmer on low heat for 40 minutes. Add the remaining ingredients, then continue to simmer for another 5 minutes, stirring to mix well. Continue on low heat to avoid burning.

Purée the soup until smooth, using an immersion blender.

Nutritional Information

Calories: 256 kcal, Fat: 17g, Carbs: 24g, Sugars: 11g, Protein: 6g, Fiber: 5g, Sodium: 772mg

Brown rice and chicken salad

Servings: 4

Ingredients

- 1 cup brown rice
- 4 tablespoons olive oil
- 14 oz skinless chicken breast, sliced vertically
- 1 cup edamame beans
- 4 tomatoes, quartered

- 2 x 4 oz cans sweetcorn, drained
- 2 red bell peppers, sliced thinly
- 1 small red onion, chopped
- 2 tablespoons honey
- Fresh parsley, finely chopped
- 2 small romaine lettuce, sliced
- 1 lemon, zest and juice

Directions

Cook brown rice in boiling water. Heat 2 tablespoons of olive oil over medium-high heat, in a non-stick pan. Cook the chicken breast for 3 minutes on each side, or until juices run clear and the chicken is cooked through. Transfer chicken onto a plate and squeeze 1 tablespoon of lemon juice. Allow the chicken to rest then, after the rice has boiled for 20 minutes, add the beans. Cook for another 5 minutes, or until the beans are cooked through, then drain. Prepare the rest of the vegetables, then serve with the rice and chicken slices. Season with fresh parsley.

Dressing (Optional)

In a large bowl, add 2 tablespoons of oil, honey, the rest of the lemon juice and lemon, zest. Whisk together. Pour the dressing onto the chicken slices. mixture and stir to combine.

Nutritional Information

Calories: 500 kcal, Fat: 15g, Carbs: 51g, Sugars: 15g, Protein: 30g, Fiber: 10g, Sodium: 350mg

Spiced lentil soup

Servings: 6

Ingredients

- 1 tablespoon extra virgin olive oil
- ¼ cup chopped onion
- ½ can chopped tomatoes
- 4 cloves garlic, chopped
- 1 large carrot, chopped
- 1 large celery stalk, chopped
- ¼ teaspoon crushed red pepper flakes, or more to taste
- ¼ teaspoon cayenne pepper, or more to taste
- salt and ground black pepper
- 6 cups water
- 4 cubes chicken bouillon
- 1 ½ cups dry lentils

Directions

In a large saucepan, heat olive oil over medium heat. Cook onion and garlic for 5 minutes, or until translucent. Stir in chopped carrot and celery stalk. Cook for 8 minutes, stirring often. Add chopped tomatoes, cayenne pepper, crushed red pepper, salt, black pepper, lentils, and chicken stock. Bring to a boil and turn down the heat, allowing the soup to simmer for about 20 minutes, or until the lentils are soft.

Nutritional Information

Calories: 235 kcal, Fat: 4g, Carbs: 35g, Sugars: 6g, Protein: 16g, Fiber: 15g, Sodium: 800mg

Kale salad with quinoa and chicken

Servings: 2

Ingredients

- 1 cup cooked quinoa
- 5 cups kale
- ½ cup shaved cucumbers
- ½ cup radishes, sliced
- ½ cup cooked brown lentils
- 2 cups cooked chicken, sliced
- ¼ cup low-sodium, low-sugar Greek salad dressing, optional.

Directions

Place chicken, kale, quinoa, lentils, radishes, and cucumbers on a large plate. Add Greek salad dressing (if desired).

Nutritional Information

Calories: 400 kcal, Fat: 10g, Carbs: 25g, Sugars: 3g, Protein: 40g, Fiber: 5g, Sodium: 400mg

Vegetable and hummus pita pockets

Servings: 1

Ingredients

- 1 whole-wheat pita bread
- 4 tablespoons hummus
- ½ cup mixed salad greens
- ½ cup roasted root vegetables (recipe below)

Roasted Root Vegetable Ingredients

- 1 ½ tablespoons apple cider vinegar
- 1 large carrot, peeled, sliced thickly into ½ inches
- 1 medium parsnip, peeled, sliced thickly into ½ inches

- 1 medium beet, peeled, thickly cut into ½-inch deep wedges
- 1/2 medium red onion, peeled, thickly cut into ½-inch deep wedges
- 1/2 medium sweet potato, cut into ¾-inch cubes
- 3 tablespoons olive oil
- 1 tablespoon fresh herbs of your choice
- ½ teaspoon salt
- ½ teaspoon ground black pepper

Directions

Preheat oven to 425 degrees. Line one baking sheet with parchment paper. Add vegetables into a large bowl and add vinegar, oil, herbs, salt, and pepper and toss to coat. Line the vegetables in a single layer on the baking sheet and bake for 30-40 minutes.

Cut the pita pocket into two. Spread 2 tablespoons of hummus on each side of the pita pocket. Add the salad greens and root vegetables in a large bowl and toss. Fill each pita half with the mix.

Nutritional Information

Calories: 400 kcal, Fat: 10 g, Carbs: 60g, Sugars: 5g, Protein: 12g, Fiber: 10g, Sodium: 800mg

Banana Whole Wheat Muffin with Tomato and Arugula Salad

Servings: 12

Ingredients for banana muffins

- 2 large bananas, mashed
- 2 large eggs
- ⅓ cup coconut oil
- ⅓ cup honey
- ⅓ cup almond milk
- 1 cup chopped walnuts
- 2 cups whole wheat flour, leveled
- ½ cup whole rolled oats
- 1 teaspoon ground cinnamon
- 1 teaspoon baking soda
- 1 teaspoon baking powder
- ½ teaspoon salt
- 1 teaspoon vanilla extract

Ingredients for tomato and arugula salad (one serving)

- 8-10 cherry tomatoes, sliced
- 1 cup arugula, washed
- 1 tablespoon olive oil
- 1 tablespoon balsamic vinegar

Directions

Preheat oven to 425°F. Line a 12-muffin pan with muffin liners. Sieve the oat flour, baking soda, baking powder, and salt into a large bowl. Add oats and then set aside. Whisk the flour, oats, cinnamon, baking soda, baking powder, and salt together in a large bowl until combined. Set aside. In another bowl, whisk together the oil, vanilla, mashed bananas, honey, milk, and eggs. Fold the dry ingredients into the wet ingredients, then add the nuts until everything is combined. Divide the batter evenly into muffin liners and bake for 20 minutes at 375 degrees. Transfer onto a wire rack to cool.

Serve tomato and arugula salad, topped with olive oil and balsamic vinegar dressing. One banana muffin on the side.

Nutritional Information

Calories: 200 kcal, Fat: 9g, Carbs: 30g, Sugars: 7g, Protein: 5g, Fiber: 3g, Sodium: 100mg

Falafel avocado wrap with garlic aioli

Servings: 3

Ingredients

- 1 can chickpeas, drained
- 3 tablespoons chickpea flour
- ½ cup spring onion
- 1 cup parsley, chopped
- 1 cup fresh cilantro, chopped
- 1 small habanero pepper, finely chopped
- 4 garlic cloves, finely chopped
- 1 teaspoon cumin
- 1 teaspoon salt
- ½ tsp cardamom
- ¼ teaspoon black pepper
- ½ teaspoon baking soda
- Olive oil for frying

Ingredients for the garlic aioli

- ½ cup low-fat mayonnaise (vegan preferred)
- 1 tablespoon lemon juice
- 1 clove garlic, minced
- ¼ teaspoon kosher salt
- 1 teaspoon extra virgin oil
- ⅓ teaspoon pepper

Directions

Add onion, herbs, chickpeas, salt, pepper, and black pepper into a food processor. Pulse until the mixture is coarse. In a large bowl, add the chickpea mixture, chickpea flour, and baking soda, then mix. Cover the bowl with a lid and keep the mixture in the fridge for an hour. Take the mixture out of the fridge, then make similar-sized falafel balls. Spritz oil on the falafel balls and bake for 25-30 minutes at 375 degrees F.

To make the garlic aioli, mix all the ingredients together.

Nutritional Information

Calories: 400 kcal, Fat: 10g, Carbs: 20g, Sugars: 5g, Protein: 7g, Fiber: 5g, Sodium: 500mg

Green salad with edamame and beets

Servings: 1

Ingredients

- 2 cups mixed salad greens, or iceberg lettuce
- 1 cup shelled edamame, thawed
- ½ cup raw beet, peeled and shredded
- 2½ tablespoons red wine vinegar
- 1 tablespoon chopped fresh cilantro

- 2 teaspoons extra-virgin olive oil
- Salt and pepper, to taste

Directions

On a large plate, arrange edamame, greens, and beet on a large plate. In another bowl, whisk together vinegar, salt and pepper, and cilantro, then drizzle over the salad.

Nutritional Information

Calories: 300 kcal, Fat: 15g, Carbs: 20g, Sugars: 4g, Protein: 20g, Fiber: 45g, Sodium: 600mg

Vegan superfood Buddha bowls with miso sauce

Servings: 4

Ingredients

- 1 cup of brown rice
- 2 cups kale, finely chopped
- 2 avocados, sliced
- 1 small butternut squash, diced
- 2 tablespoons olive oil
- Sunflower seeds, optional

For the Miso Sauce

- ¼ cup white miso paste
- ¼ cup nutritional yeast
- 4 tablespoons soy sauce
- 3 tablespoons maple syrup/honey
- 2 garlic cloves, minced
- 1 tbsp of grated fresh ginger
- 2 tbsp of lime juice
- ½ cup of avocado oil
- 2-3 tablespoons of water

Directions

Cook the brown rice, then set aside. Preheat the oven to 400 degrees F. Toss the butternut squash with olive oil, then arrange on a baking sheet and roast for 15 minutes. Turn over, then roast for another 15 minutes. Cook the kale in a separate pan for about 4 minutes, then drain. Set aside. Plate all the ingredients.

Prepare the miso sauce by placing all the ingredients together in a blender. Drizzle the sauce over the Buddha bowl. Sprinkle with sesame seeds, if desired.

Nutritional Information

Calories: 600 kcal, Fat: 32g, Carbs: 60g, Sugars: 13g, Protein: 25g, Fiber: 15g, Sodium: 1000mg

Slow cooker vegetable stew

Servings: 6

Ingredients

- 1 cup vegetable broth
- 2 large carrots, sliced thickly
- 2 medium leeks, sliced
- 1 small butternut squash, cut into 1-inch chunks
- 1 medium onion, chopped
- 2 ribs celery, sliced
- 1 cup mushrooms, sliced
- 15 oz can white beans, drained and rinsed
- 15 oz can crushed tomatoes
- ½ pound small white potatoes, rinsed and unpeeled
- 1 bay leaf

Directions

Layer all the ingredients in a 4-5 quart slow cooker. Cook on low for 5 to 7 hours, or until vegetables are tender.

Nutritional Information

Calories: 175 kcal, Fat: 2g, Carbs: 34g, Sugars: 5g, Protein: 10g, Fiber: 7g, Sodium: 400mg

Dinner Recipes

Honey garlic salmon with quinoa

Servings: 1

Ingredients

- 1 3-4oz fresh salmon
- 3 tablespoons olive oil + ¼ cup olive oil
- ½ teaspoon garlic powder
- Salt and pepper, to taste
- ½ cup carrots, sliced
- ½ cup broccoli florets
- ¼ cup onion, sliced
- 1 cup, dry quinoa
- 3 cups low-sodium chicken broth
- 2 tablespoons white balsamic vinegar

Directions

Preheat oven to 400 degrees F. Spray non-stick cooking spray on a baking pan or line the baking pan with parchment paper. Place the salmon on the baking pan, then sprinkle salt, pepper, and garlic powder on both sides. Lightly drizzle with olive oil and bake for 15-20 minutes.

While the salmon bakes, bring quinoa, onions and broccoli to boil in chicken broth, then simmer for 15 minutes, or until the liquid is fully absorbed. Add more liquid if necessary.

Mix ¼ cup olive oil with balsamic vinegar, salt, and pepper and stir to combine.

Plate quinoa, vegetables, and salmon and drizzle with balsamic vinegar sauce.

Nutritional Information

Calories: 700 kcal, Fat: 45g, Carbs: 80g, Sugars: 40g, Protein: 25g, Fiber: 5g, Sodium: 50mg

Shrimp fajitas with avocados

Servings: 3

Ingredients

- 3 tablespoons olive oil, divided
- 1 tablespoon onion powder, divided
- 6 cherry tomatoes, sliced
- 1 bag mixed salad leaves

- 2 teaspoon taco/fajita seasoning, divided
- 1 pound medium shrimp, peeled and deveined
- 2 tablespoons fresh cilantro, divided
- 6 (10 inch) grain tortillas, warmed
- 2 small avocados, sliced
- 1 tablespoon fresh cilantro
- 1 fresh lime, juiced
- Salt and pepper to taste

Directions

In a large bowl, add the sliced avocados, 1 tablespoon fresh cilantro, juice of fresh lime, 1 tablespoon of olive oil, and salt and pepper. Mix, cover and set aside. In a large skillet, heat 1 tablespoon of olive oil over medium-high heat. Add the cherry tomatoes, half the onion powder, and half the taco/fajita seasoning. Stir frequently, until tomatoes are still slightly crisp. Remove from the skillet and set aside.

Pour 1 tablespoon of olive oil into the hot skillet and add the shrimp and the remaining half of the seasoning. Add 1 tablespoon of fresh cilantro and salt and pepper and cook. Stir occasionally until the shrimp is pink and opaque. Add tomatoes back in and stir, then remove from heat. Assemble fajitas by first layering the salad leaves on the bottom of the tortillas. Add the tomatoes, followed by the shrimp, then top with the avocado salsa.

Nutritional Information

Calories: 500 kcal, Fat: 30g, Carbs: 20g, Sugars: 5g, Protein: 25g, Fiber: 5g, Sodium: 800mg

Turmeric lentil soup

Servings: 6

Ingredients

- 1 tablespoon olive oil
- 1 cup onion, chopped
- 1 large sweet potato, chopped
- 2 garlic cloves, minced
- 1 cup green or brown lentils
- 1 cup red lentils
- 1 tablespoon turmeric
- 1 teaspoon ginger
- 1 teaspoon cumin
- 4 cups vegetable broth
- 2 cups water
- 1 cup almond milk
- 1 cup spinach
- 2 teaspoons dried thyme
- 1 teaspoon lemon juice

- ½ teaspoon red pepper flakes
- Salt and pepper to taste

Directions

Heat the olive oil in a pot over medium heat. Add onions, sweet potato and garlic and sauté for about 5 minutes, until slightly softened. Season with salt, pepper, and thyme, and cook for another 2 minutes. Add lentils, turmeric, ginger, and cumin and sauté for 2 minutes, before adding the broth and water. Bring the soup to a boil, then cover and simmer for 30 minutes. Remove from heat and stir in almond milk, spinach, lemon, pepper flakes, and herbs of your choice. Stir until the spinach has wilted. Serve immediately and freeze leftovers.

Nutritional Information

Calories: 330 kcal, Fat: 5g, Carbs: 63g, Sugars: 5g, Protein: 20g, Fiber: 10g, Sodium: 500mg

Butternut squash soup

Servings: 6

Ingredients

- 3 lb butternut squash, cubed and roasted
- 2 tablespoons olive oil
- 1 ½ cups chopped onion
- 6 cups vegetable broth
- toasted pumpkin seeds, optional, to garnish
- ¼ teaspoon salt
- ⅛ teaspoon black pepper
- ⅛ tsp ground cinnamon

Directions

Add olive oil to a large pot. Over medium heat, add onion, salt, and pepper, and cook until onions turn translucent. Add the roasted butternut squash cubes. Add cinnamon and cook for 2 minutes. The cinnamon will begin to smell fragrant. Add the vegetable stock, then bring to a boil. Simmer for 2 minutes, then blend using an immersion blender. Salt and pepper to taste. Garnish with pumpkin seeds, if preferred.

Nutritional Information

Calories: 160 kcal, Fat: 5g, Carbs: 30g, Sugars: 5g, Protein: 3g, Fiber: 5g, Sodium: 230mg

Salmon and Asparagus with Lemon Butter Garlic Sauce

Servings: 4

Ingredients

- 1 lb salmon filet
- 1 pound fresh asparagus, trimmed
- ½ teaspoon ground pepper
- 3 tablespoons butter
- 2 tablespoon olive oil
- ½ tablespoon grated garlic
- 1 teaspoon grated lemon zest
- 1 tablespoon lemon juice
- ½ teaspoon salt
- ½ teaspoon ground black pepper

Directions

Preheat oven to 375 degrees F. Grease a baking sheet with oil, then place salmon on one side and asparagus on the other side. Sprinkle the salmon with salt and pepper. In a small pan, over medium heat, heat garlic, lemon zest, butter, oil and lemon juice. Drizzle the mixture onto salmon and asparagus. Bake asparagus and salmon for 15 minutes, or until salmon is cooked through.

Nutritional Information

Calories: 260 kcal, Fat: 17g, Carbs: 7g, Sugars: 3g, Protein: 27g, Fiber: 4g, Sodium: 351mg

Chickpea Avocado Salad

Servings: 4

Ingredients

- ½ cup 1 avocado
- 1 (15 oz) can chickpeas, drained and rinsed
- 10 cherry tomatoes, halved
- 2 tablespoons olive oil
- ½ lemon, juiced
- ⅓ cup parsley
- 2 cups fresh spinach, or other vegetables you like, such as shredded carrots and sliced cucumbers
- ½ teaspoon Italian seasoning
- 2 tablespoons sunflower seeds
- Salt and pepper to taste

Directions

Add the avocado, cherry tomatoes, and spinach in a large bowl. Add chopped parsley and chickpeas. Drizzle over olive oil and lemon juice. Season with salt, pepper, and Italian seasoning. Then sprinkle the sunflower seeds and serve. Store leftovers in the refrigerator, in a sealed container, for up to 3 days.

Nutritional Information

Calories: 330 kcal, Fat: 24g, Carbs: 25g, Sugars: 4g, Protein: 14g, Fiber: 15g, Sodium: 300mg

Vegetarian Niçoise Salad

Servings: 1

Ingredients

- 2 cups mixed salad greens
- 4 tablespoons lemon vinaigrette, divided
- ¼ cup steamed green beans
- ¼ cup diced cooked baby potatoes
- ¼ cup cherry tomatoes, halved
- 2 hard-boiled eggs, halved
- ½ ounce pitted Kalamata olives

Directions

Add salad greens with vinaigrette in a large bowl. Toss and plate. Add green beans, potatoes and 2 tablespoons of vinaigrette in another large bowl and toss. Layer onto salad greens. Add tomatoes, eggs, and olives.

Nutritional Information

Calories: 350 kcal, Fat: 26g, Carbs: 20 g, Sugars: 4g, Protein: 13g, Fiber: 5g, Sodium: 700mg

Vegan White Bean Chili

Servings: 6

Ingredients

- ½ cup olive oil
- 2 tbsp olive oil
- 1 medium onion, diced
- 2 medium potatoes, peeled and diced
- 4 cups vegetable broth
- 7.5 cups white kidney beans, drained and rinsed
- 2 cups corn, canned or frozen
- ½ cup cilantro, chopped
- 1 jalapeño pepper, diced and seeded
- 2 cloves garlic, minced

- ½ teaspoon thyme
- ½ teaspoon oregano
- 1 teaspoon cumin
- 1 teaspoon paprika
- 1 teaspoon chili powder
- ½ teaspoon chili flakes (optional)
- 1 lime, juiced and zested
- Salt and pepper to taste

Directions

In a large pot, over medium heat, sauté garlic, onions, and jalapeño in the olive oil for 5 minutes, or until translucent. Add the spices, broth, and potatoes, then bring to a boil. Simmer and cook for 15 minutes, or until potatoes are tender. Add beans and continue to simmer lightly for 15-20 minutes. Add corn and cilantro, then simmer for another 3 minutes. Turn off the heat and add lime juice, lime zest, chili, salt and black pepper.

Nutritional Information

Calories: 350 kcal, Fat: 3g, Carbs: 60g, Sugars: 5g, Protein: 20, Fiber: 15g, Sodium: 800mg

Open-Face Grilled Turkey Burger with Baked Sweet Potato Fries

Servings: 1

Ingredients

- 1 medium sweet potato, cut into fries
- 1 tablespoon extra virgin olive oil
- 1 ounce turkey burger pattie
- 1 oat bread burger bun
- 1 avocado, mashed
- ½ cup shredded lettuce
- 1/2 cup chopped tomatoes
- ¼ cup red onion, chopped
- Salt, pepper and garlic powder to taste

Directions

Preheat oven to 450 degrees F. Place sweet potato fries in a large bowl and add salt, pepper and garlic powder to taste. Toss and spread evenly onto a baking sheet. Bake for 30 minutes, turning occasionally.

Spray cooking spray on both sides of the turkey burger, then grill. Season with black pepper, salt, and garlic powder to taste. Top bottom of burger bun with shredded lettuce and mashed avocado. Add the patty and top with the tomatoes and red onion.

Nutritional Information

Calories: 120 kcal, Fat: 2g, Carbs: 25g, Sugars: 20g, Protein: 5g, Fiber: 4g, Sodium: 70mg

Baked Salmon Tacos

Servings: 4

Ingredients

- 4 corn tortillas, warmed
- ½ pound fresh salmon
- 1 avocado, diced
- 2 cups iceberg lettuce, shredded
- Handful of spinach leaves
- ½ lime, juiced
- 1 teaspoon olive oil
- 1 cup non-fat Greek yogurt
- 1 clove garlic, minced
- Fresh cilantro, chopped
- Salt, pepper, garlic powder and ground cumin, to taste

Directions

Preheat oven to 375 degrees F. Coat the salmon in olive oil and sprinkle both sides with salt, pepper, ground cumin, and garlic powder. Cook in the oven for 10-15 minutes or until the fish flakes easily. Roughly cut the salmon into bite sized pieces and set aside.

In a small bowl, mix the yogurt, lime juice, garlic, and cilantro together. Layer the corn tortillas with lettuce, spinach, avocado, and sauce.

Nutritional Information

Calories: 340 kcal, Fat: 18g, Carbs: 18g, Sugars: 3g, Protein: 30g, Fiber: 4g, Sodium: 500mg

30-Day Meal Plan

As you prepare these meals and plan for the weeks ahead, being the new healthiest version of yourself, feel free to switch the meals around. All recipes aid in good digestion and can be consumed in any order. Below is a suggested order based on convenience. You will notice some recipes call for more than one serving and a meal may be repeated the next day. That's because I know how busy life can get, and having already prepared meals on hand will save you a lot of time!

Tip: Freeze extra portions of the soups, stews, and muffins so they stay fresh.

Day 1

- Breakfast: Berry Kefir Smoothie
- Lunch: Brown rice and chicken salad
- Dinner: Turmeric lentil soup

Day 2

- Breakfast: Lemon blueberry muffins
- Lunch: Brown rice and chicken salad
- Dinner: Salmon tacos

Day 3

- Breakfast: Tomato and leek frittatas
- Lunch: Slow cooker vegetable stew
- Dinner: Turmeric lentil soup

Day 4

- Breakfast: Ginger and mango smoothie
- Lunch: Spiced lentil soup
- Dinner: Open-faced turkey burger with baked sweet potato fries

Day 5

- Breakfast: Peanut Butter Banana Toast
- Lunch: Vegan superfood Buddha bowls
- Dinner: Butternut squash soup

Day 6

- Breakfast: Berry kefir smoothie
- Lunch: Green salad with edamame and beets
- Dinner: Salmon and asparagus with lemon butter garlic sauce

Day 7

- Breakfast: Strawberry smoothie with chia seeds and Greek yogurt
- Lunch: Slow cooker vegetable stew
- Dinner: Shrimp fajitas with avocados

Day 8

- Breakfast: Oats with bananas, almonds and almond butter
- Lunch: Brown rice and chicken salad
- Dinner: Shrimp fajitas with avocados

Day 9

- Breakfast: Lemon blueberry muffins
- Lunch: Vegetable and hummus pita pockets
- Dinner: Honey garlic salmon with quinoa

Day 10

- Breakfast: Berry kefir smoothie
- Lunch: Vegetable and hummus pita pockets
- Dinner: Vegetarian niçoise salad

Day 11

- Breakfast: Sweet potato pancakes
- Lunch: Banana wholewheat muffins with tomato and arugula salad
- Dinner: Vegan white bean chili

Day 12

- Breakfast: Lemon blueberry muffins
- Lunch: Spiced lentil soup
- Dinner: Shrimp fajitas with avocados

Day 13

- Breakfast: Strawberry smoothie with chia seeds and Greek yogurt
- Lunch: Green salad with edamame and beets
- Dinner: Vegetarian niçoise salad

Day 14

- Breakfast: Avocado toast with poached eggs
- Lunch: Thai carrot soup
- Dinner: Honey garlic salmon with quinoa

Day 15

- Breakfast: Lemon blueberry muffins
- Lunch: Kale salad with quinoa and chicken
- Dinner: Open-faced turkey burger with baked sweet potato fries

Day 16

- Breakfast: Ginger and mango smoothie
- Lunch: Banana wholewheat muffins with tomato and arugula salad
- Dinner: Chickpea avocado salad

Day 17

- Breakfast: Tomato and leek frittatas
- Lunch: Falafel avocado wrap with garlic aioli
- Dinner: Honey garlic salmon with quinoa

Day 18

- Breakfast: Strawberry smoothie with chia seeds and Greek yogurt
- Lunch: Falafel avocado wrap with garlic aioli
- Dinner: Salmon tacos

Day 19

- Breakfast: Ginger and mango smoothie
- Lunch: Vegan superfood Buddha bowls
- Dinner: Butternut squash soup

Day 20

- Breakfast: Sweet potato pancakes
- Lunch: Vegetable and hummus pita pockets
- Dinner: Vegan white bean chili

Day 21

- Breakfast: Lemon blueberry muffins
- Lunch: Green salad with edamame and beets
- Dinner: Salmon and asparagus with lemon butter garlic sauce

Day 22

- Breakfast: Ginger and mango smoothie
- Lunch: Slow cooker vegetable stew
- Dinner: Vegetarian niçoise salad

Day 23

- Breakfast: Oats with bananas, almonds and almond butter
- Lunch: Spiced lentil soup
- Dinner: Vegetarian Niçoise salad

Day 24

- Breakfast: Avocado toast with poached eggs
- Lunch: Kale salad with quinoa and chicken
- Dinner: Turmeric lentil soup

Day 25

- Breakfast: Strawberry smoothie with chia seeds and Greek yogurt
- Lunch: Banana wholewheat muffins with tomato and arugula salad
- Dinner: Salmon and asparagus with lemon butter garlic sauce

Day 26

- Breakfast: Oats with bananas, almonds, and almond butter
- Lunch: Thai carrot soup
- Dinner: Shrimp fajitas with avocados

Day 27

- Breakfast: Ginger and mango smoothie
- Lunch: Slow cooker vegetable stew
- Dinner: Butternut squash soup

Day 28

- Breakfast: Overnight oats with berries and chia seeds
- Lunch: Vegan superfood Buddha bowls
- Dinner: Vegan white bean chili

Day 29

- Breakfast: Peanut butter banana toast
- Lunch: Falafel avocado wrap with garlic aioli
- Dinner: Chickpea avocado salad

Day 30

- Breakfast: Overnight oats with berries and chia seeds
- Lunch: Slow cooker vegetable stew
- Dinner: Honey garlic salmon with quinoa

Now that you understand how to nurture your gut to improve your digestion and reap the benefits of a healthy digestive system, it's time to tackle how the gut affects other areas of general health, starting with your hormones.

PART II

RESTORE YOUR HEALTH

4

MEET THE ESTROBOLOME: UNDERSTANDING GUT HEALTH AND HORMONES

> *"When gut health isn't optimal, hormones become imbalanced."*
>
> — LEIGH ANN SCOTT, M.D.

By now, you are probably feeling good, eating healthy, exercising regularly, just being awesome! You may have started noticing changes in your body, like a flatter stomach, glowing skin and increased energy! You may just generally be feeling as though it's good to be alive!

Now it's time to talk about another important factor that influences our gut health: hormones. Many of my clients are shocked when I share with them how their hormones actually determine whether or not they can achieve that flat tummy. Like your diet and exercise, hormones are critical to what goes on not just in our gut, but in all other parts of our body. In this chapter, I will give you tips on how to maintain and improve your hormone balance, so you can stay looking amazing and feeling great!

METABOLIZING ESTROGEN: MEET ESTROBOLOME

What is estrobolome, and why does it make the red squiggly line appear whenever you type it? I think scientists just like to give things complicated names to mess with us. The unsexy name, estrobolome, actually fits because it is a collection of decidedly unsexy bacteria in our guts that regulate our estrogen levels. Why do we need to pay particular attention to estrobolome out of all the billions of bacteria in our guts? Well, because estrogen is a ridiculously important hormone in women's (and men's) bodies. It regulates so many functions, most of which we take for granted. (This is one of the reasons why menopause is so challenging - because you have to get used to lower levels of estrogen all of a sudden, which changes the way your entire body operates.)

Hence, it's safe to say that estrobolome, the guys who regulate your body's regulator, are critical to your health. They are like the really important CIA guys, in stereotypical black sunglasses and suits, closely regulating the estrogen activity in your body. It may be stereotypical, but when you give them the tools they need to do their job well (i.e., good diet and regular exercise), these CIA agents become super muscular superheroes, just punching their way to a healthy you!

Estrogen affects your bone health, sex drive, cognitive health, the way your heart functions, your skin's health, and so much more. If you have too much estrogen in your body, you could gain weight, develop anxiety or depression, and even suffer from constant exhaustion. Conversely, with the right amount of estrobolome, your body is able to properly synthesize the enzyme called beta-glucuronidase. Beta-glucuronidase breaks down complex carbohydrates and helps you absorb your micronutrients. It also prevents your body from reabsorbing too much estrogen which, if allowed to happen, spikes your estrogen levels to dangerous highs (known as estrogen dominance). It also does the opposite, preventing your estrogen levels from getting too low (known as estrogen deficiency). This entire process is known as estrogen metabolism.

The process of estrogen metabolism works like this. Your body cycles estrogen in every part so that those body parts that need estrogen can gobble some up. Just imagine the cells in your hair gobbling up some estrogen like Mr. Pacman gobbles up those white balls (which I like to imagine are dumplings). Once your body completes this process, it sends any excess estrogen to your liver. There, it is broken down into what is known as "estrogen metabolite." Some of the estrogen will be placed in the pile meant for reabsorption, and some will be placed in the pile for elimination. Your liver is basically sorting its estrogen laundry at this stage. Then it sends it to the laundromat: your intestines. At the laundromat, the estrogen marked "eliminated" is eliminated through your feces. The ones marked reabsorbed are reabsorbed.

What we can say, therefore, is that beta-glucuronidase is the Goldilocks of your body's estrogen levels, making sure that your estrogen levels are just right! Together, your estrogen's Goldilocks and superhero CIA agents work hand in hand to regulate estrogen to a happy medium. Maybe I need to have my imagination checked, but you get the picture. If you eat well, there will be less estrogen to be reabsorbed and more estrobolome to produce enough beta-glucuronidase to do its job regulating. It's a health cycle that all begins in your gut!

WHY ESTROGEN?

Let's dive a bit deeper into estrogen and how it affects our gut health. Estrogen is notoriously known as the "female" hormone because it plays a crucial role in the cardiovascular, reproductive, skeletal, and central nervous systems. You wouldn't believe how many parts of your body estrogen manages. For example, estrogen is what prevents women from developing osteoporosis, insulin insensitivity (prediabetes and diabetes), and metabolic diseases. It regulates your energy levels which is what gives you the motivation you need to exercise or prepare healthy meals.

When you have dysbiosis, it means your Goldilocks (your beta-glucuronidase) will either fall asleep in a bed that's too hard or too soft. If this leads to estrogen dominance, you become more at risk of breast cancer, ovarian cancer, and uterine cancer. In addition, dysbiosis leads to inflammation in your body, which is another cause of cancer. Estrogen imbalance is also typically associated with other chronic illnesses, namely obesity and chronic liver diseases.

Your diet affects how much estrobolome is in your gut. By now, you know the drill! The healthier your diet, the more you produce the right conditions for estrobolome to thrive! For example, people on a vegetarian, plant-based, and high-fiber diet have a better "just right" amount of estrogen than people on a higher fat or higher protein diet. In fact, vegetarian women have fewer incidences of breast cancer, as opposed to women who eat meat. This is partly because vegetarian women excrete two to three times more estrogen than omnivorous women, meaning that they don't reabsorb excess hormones.

You can improve conditions for your estrobolome to thrive by eating foods high in unsaturated fats, such as olive oil, cod liver oil, and homemade nut butters. Getting a healthy amount of protein from low-dairy products, lean meats, and legumes. Adding foods with antioxidants and anti-inflammatory properties to your diet. Incorporating fresh and dried herbs in your diet, such as ginger, sumac, basil, turmeric, and paprika. Eat plenty of spices. Spices like black pepper, cinnamon, and cayenne pepper promote the growth of healthy bacteria. Eating foods high in fiber. Although we've discussed this before, it's worth repeating, since research shows that just increasing your fiber intake by 10 grams a day reduces your chance of developing breast cancer by 7%. Drinking blackcurrant tea, or including fresh/frozen blackcurrants in your diet. They allow your beta-glucuronidase to work at optimal levels! Eating foods high in vitamin A, like carrots, spinach, sweet potatoes, and red bell peppers. As well as incorporating foods high in vitamin D3, like oatmeal, eggs, and mushrooms. Choosing foods with plenty of phytoestrogens. Phytoestrogens are plant estrogens that are so similar to human estrogens that they work in our bodies when we ingest them. They block estrogen receptors in our body when our estrogen levels get too high, thereby protecting you from excessive estrogen exposure. Leafy greens, peaches, garlic, soy, nuts, cruciferous vegetables, legumes, and some seeds, such as ground flax seeds, are great sources of phytoestrogens. Speaking with your doctor if you are on birth control, as it affects your estrogen levels, as well as the microbial balance in your intestines. Avoiding Calcium-D-Glucarate supplements because they act as beta-glucuronidase inhibitors.

These foods and medicines significantly lower your chances of developing the chronic conditions discussed above. Likewise, they help reduce your chances of developing the following health conditions:

- Premenstrual symptoms, e.g., migraines, bloating, increased period pain, and heavy periods
- Polycystic ovary syndrome (PCOS)
- Cystic breast pain
- Endometriosis
- Infertility

- Mood disturbance
- Low libido
- Insomnia

ESTROBOLOME AND GUT HEALTH

Your body is just one big interconnected machine. Anything that happens to one part directly or indirectly affects other parts. Before we move on to other ways our guts affect our bodies, let's examine another part of our estrobolome-health connection.

A healthy microflora is like a healthy garden. It has a wide diversity of organisms and is bursting with life that is beneficial to the earth. If you are familiar with gardening, you know that the best way to make your garden thrive is to position plants in such a way that they benefit each other. You also keep out plants and pests that are decidedly not beneficial to your plants.

An unhealthy gut is like an unhealthy garden, with plants positioned wherever, so that they never thrive, and pests and weeds grow all over the place. If you have too many unhealthy bacteria in your estrobolome, your beta-glucuronidase will malfunction and allow excess estrogen to be reabsorbed into your body. This is clearly bad news. Likewise, you also need a healthy biodiversity if you want to promote a healthy balance of beta-glucuronidase activity. With a low microfloral biodiversity, your estrobolome won't be able to convert estrogen, whether in its original form or as phytoestrogens. This then leads to the opposite, with less estrogen absorbed by your body.

We've focused mainly on estrogen in this chapter, but there are other just as important hormones in your body, all connected to your gut health, such as testosterone (our sex hormone), melatonin (which helps us sleep), and cortisol (our stress-reducing hormone). They all rely on a healthy gut microbiota to stay balanced. And they are all so finely tuned to your gut health that even a week of adding high sugar juice to your diet can cause them to become imbalanced. I think we take for granted just how delicate our gut ecosystem is, and how it affects everything in our lives. For example, I have noticed that if I eat healthy in the two weeks leading up to my period, I have a cramp-free, bloat-free, and light period. If I eat a few desserts the week before, however, some of these symptoms reappear.

Before making food, fitness, and health choices, it is always important to remember that you need to keep your hormones in balance through your gut health. This promotes good health by helping your body to synthesize (produce) the hormones it needs, keeping your immune system healthy, and improving how much nutrients you absorb from your food, thereby making you a healthier person in general.

GUT HEALTH AND HORMONAL BALANCE

Your hormones are your body's messengers, controlling a significant part of your body's processes. They are those old-fashioned telegram delivery services you see when you watch fancy old British shows. However, they don't just deliver messages per se, as much as they deliver commands. When you're hungry, leptin commands that you be informed that it's time to eat some salad. Once you get full, ghrelin kicks in to tell you that you can stop eating now. When it's nighttime, melatonin commands your body to make you sleepy, so you can rest and give your body a chance to heal itself.

These messages never stop, even when you're asleep. They are like train tracks, keeping the entire community that is your body running effectively. If you've ever experienced needing to travel by train during a rail strike, you know how important punctual trains are. Or, for a more modern example, think of if we were all unable to send each other emails or any other form of electronic messages for an entire week. Every single aspect of our lives will collapse because we rely on these messages to keep the world going. That's how important your hormones are. And, because every part of your body is interconnected and interdependent on the other, even if one hormone is not able to function properly, it ends up affecting every other part of your ecosystem.

If your hormones are like the train tracks, then your endocrine system is the rail company itself. They are in charge of these tracks, directing them to their destinations on time. Your endocrine system is made up of your hormones and most of the tissue that is in charge of creating and releasing these hormones. Some of the bodily processes that your hormones control include:

- Reproduction
- Metabolism
- Sexual function
- Homeostasis (constant internal harmony)
- Growth and development
- Sleep-wake consumers
- Mood

In recent years, scientists are discovering that your gut microbiome plays a central role in this system, acting as a sort of "CEO" of your endocrine system. It produces your hormones (alongside your adrenal glands and ovaries), and it decides how much of each hormone to produce and release. Furthermore, your microflora is the CEO of nearly all the hormones in your body. In case you haven't gotten it yet, these microorganisms essentially run things!

As well as your gut-estrobolome balance, dysbiosis affects the following hormones:

Thyroid

This can lead to hyperthyroidism, with symptoms such as dry skin, weight gain, constipation, sensitivity to cold, and poor memory.

Melatonin

Your body cannot produce melatonin without plenty of serotonin. (Serotonin is a mood-regulating hormone). Since more than 90% of our serotonin is produced in our gut, people who have an unhealthy gut will often suffer from sleep problems.

Cortisol, Epinephrine, and Norepinephrine

These hormones are released when your body feels as though it's in danger, or whenever you feel anxious or stressed. They protect you by keeping you hyper-vigilant and high-strung. Being constantly hyper-vigilant is not good for your health. It puts too much strain on your heart, it can lead to high blood pressure, and it triggers gut imbalance. To make matters worse, if you have consistently high levels of stress hormones, research suggests that this can trigger harmful gene expression in some microbes in your gut.

As with estrogen, you can have an imbalance of other hormones. Sometimes, hormonal imbalances involve just one hormone while other times, it involves more than one. In many cases, even slightly elevated or lowered levels of one hormone can cause major changes in your bodily processes, easily leading to health conditions and even chronic diseases. That's why our gut health is so important because our gut essentially acts as the center of our entire health and wellness. As Dr. Karen Wallace argues: "This gut-hormone connection proves to me that gut health is again at the root of many health concerns."

HEALTHY HORMONES

Some great ways to promote hormone balance are insuring you are eating five servings of fruit and vegetables daily. As well as eating very colorful fruits and vegetables, as these are typically the healthiest for you. Taking 1 gram of L-glutamine daily can cut down on your sugar cravings. As we have previously discussed, sugar is one of the worst foods to consume. It directly feeds the bad bacteria in your gut. As these bacteria get stronger, they actually send messages to your brain to increase your sugar cravings so that you can continue to feed them. (They are pretty devious!) You can try replacing sugar with healthier artificial sweeteners, such as Stevia. Taking 200-400 mcg of chromium daily helps make your insulin receptor much more sensitive, which improves your body's capacity to burn carbs effectively. Try avoiding alcohol. Alcohol affects estrogen metabolism, causing an almost immediate hormonal imbalance in your body. It elevates estrogen levels in your blood, leading to estrogen dominance. If you want to drink alcohol, stick to moderate amounts of red wine. Red wine contains resveratrol, which is a phytoestrogen. Drink plenty of water. There's a reason people with gorgeous skin often tend to drink loads of water. Water quickly eliminates all the waste from your body. You can also swap water for decaf, green tea, decaf black tea, and other forms of herbal or spice teas. Have snacks throughout your day if you start to feel hungry between meals. Our mood and blood sugar naturally drop when we start to get hungry. Feed the beast! If you have a snack high in protein or fat, it stops you from overeating at night. Try not to eat too much at night. Our metabolic rate actually peaks around noon every day, so any food you eat after that time is more likely to be stored as fat. Avoid skipping meals or being on severe calorie-deficit diets.

This lowers your metabolic rate, causing weight gain. Ensure you are eating breakfast every day. Breakfast kick-starts your metabolism. Try using the "cupped hand" method for plating. If you cup both your hands together out in front of you, that is how big your stomach is. Try not to go over this limit when you have meals and snacks. That way, you give your body a chance to effectively and quickly digest your food, promoting your metabolic rate. The more you eat in one go, the more energy, time, and resources your body takes to digest. Like any ecosystem (or even any machine) it's best not to overload your digestive system with too much food at once.

Consume fat alongside low glycaemic index carbs. Low glycaemic index carbohydrates are carbs that do not raise your blood sugar and insulin levels immediately after consumption. As a result, they are great for people with diabetes. For prediabetic people or people who do not have diabetes, they also prevent you from developing diabetes. When you consume fat alongside low GI carbs, insulin is not secreted, meaning that it is also not stored as fat. (This tip doesn't work if you are already overproducing insulin or if you eat excessively during meals). Examples of low GI carbs include chickpeas, peanuts, soybeans, tomatoes, black beans, yogurt, and wild rice. Eating a healthy source of fat with every meal, such as olive oil, nut butter, avocados, or seeds, will aid in hormone regulation. They also enable hormone production. Choosing the right household and beauty products is a must. You want to use paraben- and phthalate-free household and beauty products and BPA-free plastics. These chemicals disrupt our hormones, leading to hormonal imbalance.

Now that you understand that different lifestyle factors can throw off your hormonal paradise, which negatively affects your gut health, there is still so much more to learn. A proper gut-healthy diet doesn't just help balance hormones. It can also slow down the aging process as well. Let's move on to find out more!

5

FOOD AS A TIME MACHINE: EATING YOUR WAY TO A YOUNGER YOU

> *"The food you eat can either be the safest and most powerful form of medicine or the slowest form of poison."*
>
> — ANN WIGMORE

Did you know that food has anti-aging benefits? It's why people who follow a healthy diet typically tend to age slower than people who eat less healthily. In scientific terms, this is known as the difference between your chronological age and your biological age. Basically, two people could be the same age (chronological age) but one could actually be younger (biological age). That's right! From now on, it's OK to list yourself as ten years younger on your dating profile because technically, you might be!

So, what exactly are chronological age and biological age?

WHAT'S YOUR REAL AGE?

Your chronological age is the age according to your passport. That is, simply, the amount of years that have passed since the day you were introduced to this world. You can't change this age, but you can change your biological age, which is how much your body has actually aged since birth. Biological age is affected by your chronological age, your diet/nutrition, your lifestyle, your genes, and your health history, for example, if you have any diseases or health conditions.

Essentially, our cells take a lot of oxidative damage on a regular basis. The more oxidative stress your cells encounter, the faster they age. It's why people who stay out of the sun keep their youthful skin much longer than people who are in the sun all the time without sun protection. The sun causes oxidative damage to our skin, leading to tans, sunburn and, in extreme cases, skin cancer. In the same way, oxidative damage is being done inside you, caused by things such as your diet, how quickly your body fights against oxidative stress, diseases, and so on.

Not only will all the information you've learned in previous chapters keep you healthy and fit, it will also slow down your aging process. Likewise, the less you follow this advice, the quicker you will age. You heard that right! Some people have a biological age much higher than their chronological age. If this doesn't motivate you to make yourself a cup of green tea, I don't know what will!

As well as the tips in previous chapters, there are also two more things you should know about reducing your biological age.

Your body shape

Your body shape is determined by the way your body distributes fat, including your waist circumference and your waist-to-hip ratio. People with pear shapes have a smaller waist, since their fat accumulates in their thighs and hips. A pear shape is considered a healthier body shape to have because fat does not accumulate around the waist and stomach. This is in contrast to the apple shape, which causes fat to accumulate around the waist and stomach, increasing your likelihood of developing breast cancer and heart disease. If you have an apple shape, you may have to workout harder and pay closer attention to your diet to ensure that you are not storing fat in your waist or stomach. It's annoying and totally unfair!

Foods with low glycemic indexes

The glycemic index of food tells you how quickly particular foods raise your blood sugar (as we discussed in Chapter Four). Foods with low glycemic indexes don't raise your blood sugar rapidly, lessening your chances of developing health conditions, such as diabetes. This also lessens your chance of biologically aging too quickly. Foods with moderate or high glycemic indexes raise your blood sugar quickly, increasing your chances of not only diabetes, but also problems with your muscles, organs, and bones.

Foods with low glycemic indexes include:

- Soya bread
- Mixed grain bread
- Rolled oats
- Porridge
- Most vegetables
- Legumes
- Cashew nuts
- Brown rice

- Whole milk
- Skimmed milk
- Soy milk

Foods with moderate glycemic indexes include:

- Mangos
- Bananas
- Raisins
- Papaya
- Basmati rice
- Beetroot
- Honey

Foods with high glycemic indexes include:

- Watermelon
- Dates
- White rice
- Potatoes
- Pumpkin
- Parsnips
- Processed foods

Other causes of oxidative damage can be:

- Pollution
- Some pesticides and household cleaners
- The ozone
- Radiation
- A diet high in sugar and fat
- Too much alcohol consumption
- Overeating
- Not giving yourself enough time between meals

One common way to prevent oxidative stress is to eat a lot of antioxidants-containing foods. This is easy to achieve if you eat your recommended five fruits and vegetables daily. Other great sources of antioxidants are:

- Garlic
- Cinnamon
- Turmeric
- Onion
- Melatonin
- Green tea
- Vitamin C
- Vitamin E
- Fish
- Nuts

HEALTHY AGING

Healthy aging simply means aging well, whilst still keeping your functional ability. For instance, being able to move your body well, eat a nutritious, fibrous meal, or go for a run is considered healthy aging. Sure, when you're twenty, it's typically easier to do all this with just as much ease as breathing. As you chronologically age, however, your body starts to see wear and tear. If you stay healthy (by following all the advice in this book), then you stay biologically younger, meaning that you are aging healthily.

Another 100% research-backed way to prove you are aging healthily is by doing "the grunt test." Here's how to do it:

1. Sit on a chair and get comfortable.
2. After about twenty minutes, try to stand up.

If you let out a huge grunt while attempting to stand up, you are now officially old enough to begin shopping around for the best denture cream in town. Okay, so maybe I made that one up, but you catch my drift.

Alternatively, you can stay healthy through tried and tested methods discussed in this book. Healthy aging doesn't just encompass the grunt test. It also involves extending your life, preventing chronic diseases, and limiting weaknesses, many of which tend to show up as we age. Let's take osteoporosis as an example. Women who exercise a lot reduce their risk of osteoporosis as they age. This, in turn, prevents them from breaking their bones if they suffer a trip or a fall in older age. In this case, a nasty cycle has been limited severely by simply exercising often. Essentially, you don't have to just accept that getting older comes with chronic illness, a reduction of life quality, and an increased likelihood of other degenerative conditions. By making healthy choices, you can significantly reduce your chances of these happening to you.

In fact, research has shown that women add, on average, fourteen years to their lifespan when they prioritize a healthy living lifestyle, while men gain, on average, twelve years.

Some other great tips for healthy aging include living a cigarette-free life, sleeping for 7-9 hours each night, having a healthy social network to support you through life's stresses, maintaining strong social ties with your family and your community, and getting annual medical checkups to spot health problems before they become serious.

MANAGING YOUR BIOLOGICAL AGE WITH FOOD

When my clients ask me what foods to eat for anti-aging, the first thing I ask them is why they want an anti-aging diet. Do they want an anti-aging diet because they want to look youthful forever, or do they want an anti-aging diet because they want to stay healthy and strong for as long as possible? There is a clear difference between the two. No matter what advertisers tell you, nobody is going to look twenty forever! All my clients are beautiful, and I mean that. You don't have to fall for the lie that you need to look incredibly young to be a hottie. When women fall into this mindset, it can cause severe mental damage and emotional distress.

Instead, eating for anti-aging is better when you have a healthy eating mindset: you eat well so that you can live a long, happy, healthy life, spending quality time with family and friends, without being limited by illness and health conditions. Sure, it's nice to look good, but this is secondary compared to actually being healthy and feeling good. Plus, when you feel good, you look good, i.e., when you prioritize healthy habits, it actually starts to show on the outside.

WHAT ARE TELOMERES? AND WHAT DO THEY HAVE TO DO WITH AGING?

Telomeres are the key to aging, but what are they? They work as a sort of aglet for your DNA. Aglets are those plastic roll things on the ends of your shoelaces that prevent your shoelaces from fraying and getting destroyed. Telomeres do the same job. They prevent your DNA strands from becoming frayed (and also from sticking to each other), allowing your DNA to work efficiently. Our DNA is in each and every one of our cells, meaning there are telomeres in every part of your body. Since our bodies make new cells by copying old ones (so that they can keep the same DNA, not because it's lazy), telomeres are also copied. The bad part is that the telomeres in each cell gets shorter every time the cell copies itself. After a while, the telomere becomes too short. When this happens, the cell ages and doesn't work as well. The cell can no longer copy itself and so it becomes inactive and dies.

This entire process is associated with aging, cancer and even death. The length of your telomeres gives a pretty good indication of your biological age because telomeres are not shortened by just aging. They are also shortened by stress, obesity, not exercising, smoking and a poor diet. I imagine it's why presidents often look so fresh and healthy just before inauguration but then look like they aged twenty years after just two years in office. All the stress of leading a country shortens their telomeres at alarming speeds, causing them to age biologically even faster than their chronological age in many cases.

The longer your telomeres, the less likely you are to develop a disease, and the slower you age. One of the best ways to keep your telomeres from shortening is to eat a diet high in folate, antioxidants (i.e., selenium, vitamin C, and vitamin E), vitamin D, and omega-3 fatty acids.

Sources of folate include:

- Beans
- Lentils
- Fortified cereals
- Fortified/enriched rice
- Fortified/enriched breads and grains
- Dark leafy green vegetables

Sources of omega-3 fatty acids include:

- Fatty fish (tuna, salmon and mackerel)
- (Ground) flax seeds
- Nuts
- Vegetable oils (soy, canola and flaxseed)

- Green leafy vegetables
- Lentils
- Algae

Sources of vitamin D include:

- Mushrooms
- Egg yolks
- Cheese
- Dairy products
- Fatty fish (tuna, salmon and mackerel)
- Sunshine

Sources of vitamin C include:

- Citrus fruits and juices
- Tomatoes
- Strawberries
- Cantaloupe
- Green leafy vegetables
- Potatoes

Sources of vitamin E include:

- Vegetable oils
- Nuts
- Seeds

Sources of selenium include:

- Dairy products
- Rice
- Grain products
- Seafood
- Brazil nuts
- Beef
- Poultry

FIGHTING INFLAMMAGING

Telomeres, inflammaging, aglet... is this a book about gut health or are we in the National Spelling Bee contest? Speaking of questions, did you know that only about 20% - 25% of our aging is down to genetics? The rest is down to epigenetics. I know. I know! I just threw in another new word! I won't go into the deep science of epigenetics except to say that it simply refers to how lifestyle, food, exercise, and all other choices in life affect the way our genes act. So, if you make positive choices often, your genes will also tend to act positively, including making you as healthy as a prize-winning horse and promoting healthy aging. Neigh way! That's awesome!

Here's what Dr. Sara Gottfried writes about epigenetics and healthy aging: "The fact is that scientists have found new ways for us to take control of our genes. For example, the naughty aging genes usually associated with fat and wrinkles can be altered with diet, exercise, and other lifestyle choices. Simply put, by turning your good genes on and your bad genes off, you can actually prevent aging - no matter how old you are."

Now that we know what epigenetics is, what's inflammaging? Inflammation can be a very deadly immune response that our body relies on. When our bodies notice things like infections or injuries, our immune system kicks into badass mode to fight off the bad guys and heal you. That's why you feel like crap when you are ill. Your immune system has kicked into overdrive in an attempt to heal you. Inflammation in small doses is OK. It's effective. However, when you begin to go through chronic inflammation (i.e., your body constantly being in a state of inflammation), this can easily shorten your telomeres. Inflammation leads to aging, hence we get the term: "inflammaging."

Research has shown that most chronic illnesses today, be it diabetes, Alzheimer's disease, hypertension, heart disease, or cancer, all stem from chronic inflammation. These health conditions listed account for half of all the deaths we see worldwide today. That means that inflammation is literally killing us. You don't have to resign yourself to this fate, however because there are ways to defeat inflammaging, namely:

- Eating an antioxidant-rich diet
- Eating a plant-rich diet, packed with fruits, vegetables and whole grains
- Eating a Mediterranean-rich diet
- Avoiding red meat and processed meat
- Eating 1-2 servings of fish weekly
- Avoiding refined (white) carbs
- Avoiding food with added sugars
- Avoiding extra processed foods, like chips
- Cutting back on excessive salt
- Eating food rich in omega-3 fatty acids
- Eating plenty of berries
- Regularly drinking tea, especially green tea
- Eating plenty of lentils, soy and leaves
- Eating plenty of cruciferous vegetables, such as cabbage, brussel sprouts, broccoli, collards and cauliflower

DE-STRESS DIARIES

Stress is a jerk! According to research on the effects of stress on our health, stress ages you, takes years off of your life span, increases your likelihood of getting sick and causes you to neglect your health and your well-being. Dr. Johnny Bowen writes that: "Stress is probably the single most potent enemy of longevity on the planet. [It] can and will shorten your life". In fact, according to Dr. Bowden, stress, along with inflammation and free radicals, are among the four horsemen of aging.

Have you ever looked at photographs of people from before the 1950s and been shocked to find out that the grandparent-looking people in the photograph are actually in their twenties? Well, not to bore you with a history lesson but, before World War Two, life was quite different, and people were under tremendous amounts of stress. It's no surprise many people died much younger back in those days too.

Stress makes you fall ill more often because it weakens your immune system. As we get older, our immune system naturally becomes less resilient, partially due to stress (remember when I said stress is a jerk?). This is why healthy aging is paramount for improving your lifespan and your quality of life.

When you are stressed, you also have to watch out for that pesky stress hormone, cortisol. Cortisol can actually damage your brain and cause hormonal imbalances. Likewise, it causes insulin imbalance and makes you store belly fat. What a splendid hormone! And if you think that's bad enough, you clearly do not realize that cortisol and stress can cause the following bodily issues; acne, under-eye bags (from a lack of sleep), rashes, wrinkles, dry skin, hair loss, graying hair, sore lips, face flushing, and tooth damage.

I wish I had a magic wand I could wave to make all the sources of your stress go away but, alas (!) my magic wand is currently in the shop for repairs. In the meantime, practice every single health advice given to you in this book to help you reduce stress. The more you practice them, the more you find out which ones your body responds most positively to. For instance, I once had a client who would spend 30 minutes on high speed on the stair climber. She said it helped her to let go of the stress of being a mother to four rambunctious children. On the plus side, her butt was the butt of gods! I had another client who hated the stair master but found that she could deal with the stresses of her day much better if she ate plenty of spinach and berries in her daily diet. Her skin was always dewy, like a glazed donut. The point is, find what works the best for you, but continue to also use as many techniques for reducing stress as you can. This brings me to the final point of this chapter: using journaling (brain dumping) as a stress-management technique.

JOURNALING

Journaling is a beautiful method for relieving stress. It's sort of like sharing your private and innermost thoughts with a trained therapist or a close friend, except this friend is a piece of paper. It allows you to release all the tension and stress you've been carrying by sharing with a non-judgemental, listening ear.

The human mind loves to share. We feel better when we communicate how we are feeling, what we are thinking, our memories, and so on. Journaling is particularly effective for helping you to jot down your negative emotions and put an objective distance between yourself and your emotions. Imagine carrying a heavy rock. These are your negative emotions. Then, imagine being able to put the rock down and take a much-needed break. Then, after you are rested and have spent some time away from it, you can come back to the rock to inspect it more objectively.

Indeed, research has shown that not only does journaling reduce stress levels, it actually reduces the rate of stress-related doctor visits that you have, lowers your blood pressure, improves your mood and keeps you healthy and well. When you write down your emotions, you're also able to process it within a safe and contained space. You will find that, the more you journal, the more you're able to process distressing, overwhelming emotions. In time, this will also help you to deal with overwhelming experiences with more resilience. All these, put together, prevent your telomeres from shortening, ultimately leading to healthy aging.

Don't get too hung up on the word "journaling." It does sound very formal, as though you're supposed to dip your quill into a pot of ink and start with the words: "Oh, verily, dear sir! Upon the moors of Telomereshire!" You really don't need to write formally, making sure everything is neat and presentable. You can just have a brain dump, dumping whatever is on your mind on a piece of paper. The effects are the same. What's important is pouring out what's going on inside of you to relieve your stress.

Here are some journaling prompts to get you started the next time you want to do a brain dump:

1. I may be stressed and anxious about things going on in my life, but I can still practice gratitude for ____.
2. Right now, I am going through the following challenges _______. However, I feel happy because I have the support of ____ , meaning that I can learn ____ from these challenges.

3. These past experiences ____ were traumatic/difficult for me, but I am strong enough to explore the pain they caused and what I learned from these experiences.
4. My inner critic might be telling me _____ but I remind myself of my past accomplishments, my skills, my qualifications and my strengths, such as _____.
5. My body feels like ____ at the moment. I feel the following physical sensations ____. I think I may be feeling these sensations because ____.
6. _____ is stressing me out. To handle my stress, I ____. Are these coping mechanisms working well for me or could I replace them with healthier coping mechanisms?
7. I need ____ to feel safe during stressful times in my life. I need to ____ to give myself this sense of safety.
8. What values do I live by? If I give it deep thought, my five most important values are _____ These values are important to me because _____ I ensure these values align with my life by _____ Some ways my actions do not align with these values are _____ because _____.
9. I least like these five things about my life _____. I will do _____ to change these things.

10. ____ treated me like this. It makes me feel like ____ because ____.

Food can de-age or slow down biological aging. If that's not a great reason to eat healthily, I don't know what is. I mean, who would you rather be? The older person grunting loudly as you attempt to stand up from a chair or the older person doing parkour on the weekends because you feel great and have no health issues holding you back? To be the latter, you have to put in the work and effort. However, since the work and effort involve eating delicious antioxidant-rich and anti-inflammatory food... I think you can manage!

6

HACKED: 15 TIPS & TRICKS TO KEEPING YOUR GUT HEALTHY

> *"If you ask what is the single most important key to longevity, I would have to say it is avoiding worry, stress and tension. And if you didn't ask me, I'd still have to say it."*
>
> — GEORGE BURNS

Food is medicine, life, health, and well-being for us. The one thing I don't want you to do is to begin your journey healing your gut health with the mentality that food is the enemy. On the contrary, it's just the way our food practices have developed in the last hundred years or so that's bad. Think back to the last time you opted to have dessert after a meal. Full of sugar, fat, salt, and maybe carbs, it must have tasted amazing!

However, even just a hundred years ago, most people wouldn't eat like this. This decadent style of eating was only reserved for the ultra-wealthy back then. If you go back even further in history, even the rich did not eat like that because we still relied on preparing food in a more natural way. Without access to cheap and plentiful seed oils, people weren't frying their chicken every two business days, and you actually had to work hard and put some physical fitness work in if you wanted to prepare something as simple as bread (as opposed to just driving to the store to buy a simple, nutrient-free white loaf).

The way we eat has changed so drastically in the last hundred years or so that most of us have to relearn what came naturally to our grandmothers and great-grandmothers: eating for life and health. This is why the diet craze of the last few decades has always failed: it's not simply about eating like a rabbit every day. It's about your mindset. Once you change how you understand food and begin to see it as a tool to keep you healthy and happy - not one meant to keep you in an addicted state of lethargy - then you begin to make wise choices. You begin to happily make good choices out of a sense of love for your body, believing that your body deserves the best. Your healthy choices, in turn, bring you mental and emotional satisfaction, keeping you away from trying to gain this satisfaction from unhealthy choices. And when you do occasionally reach for the candy bar or the extra creamy blueberry cheesecake, you do so just to give yourself a rare treat. Plus, you'll be feeling too good, too full, too satiated, and too content from your positive lifestyle choices, that you'll naturally reach for unhealthy foods less and less. Put simply, taking care of your gut health is the beginning of a healthy cycle that puts your health at the forefront of every decision you make. By taking care of your gut health, you love yourself!

In this relatively simple chapter, you will learn about 15 gut health hacks that you can easily incorporate into your lifestyle. Think of it as a condensed summary of what we've discussed in the previous chapters. With these hacks, the advice from the previous chapters has been simplified and boiled down to the basics. That way, you don't have any excuses for not loving yourself and taking care of your health. You don't necessarily have to sign up for your local parkour group, but you can still incorporate these 15 hacks into your daily routine.

1. DON'T WAIT, HYDRATE!

As we've already discussed, people who drink plenty of water tend to look amazing. Water is one of the cheapest essentials for staying healthy, and it's everywhere! So, if you're not staying hydrated, then we need to have a serious talk about your dedication to your gut health. Water is also pretty chill and easygoing. The rules are pretty simple: just drink regularly throughout your day. You will know if you are well-hydrated if your urine is a light yellow color.

You can also try this tip for improving gut health: drink plenty of water in the morning when you first wake up. I guarantee it will keep you regular. If you want to spice it up, add a tablespoon of lemon per cup or, to really feel smug about how healthy you are, add some cucumbers, mint leaves, lemons, green tea bags, and any other fruits you want to a large bottle of water. Leave it in the fridge overnight and then drink in the morning.

Another tip is to drink water before eating. This prevents you from overeating and overloading your digestive system. People have different water needs based on their lifestyles, so it's impossible to say how much water you need daily. Aim to drink at least eight glasses daily at regular intervals. As you exercise regularly and add more whole grains, lentils, and fiber to your diet, your water intake should also increase because these lifestyle choices cause your body's water needs to increase.

2. LIGHTS OUT

You want your telomeres not to shorten, right? Get enough sleep. Sleep is so important for us that everything in our bodies starts to break down when we are not getting enough - including our gut health. Getting an adequate amount of sleep (7-9 hours a day) greatly reduces your stress. There is a stress hormone known as epinephrine. If you are not getting enough sleep, epinephrine empowers your gut bacteria to multiply. Then, the gut bacteria begin to line your intestinal walls, causing inflammation. It's just a horrible cycle that puts way too much pressure on your telomeres.

If you find it difficult to sleep, try a nighttime yoga or meditation routine. I like lighting scented candles, drinking some relaxing chamomile tea, and doing a gentle bedtime yoga routine each night. Any bacteria in my gut have no chance against my calming nighttime routine.

3. EAT THE RAINBOW

The more colorful your diet, the more polyphenols you're ingesting. You're literally feeding your healthy gut bacteria with their favorite food so they grow big and tall!

4. KEEP MOVING

People who live a more sedentary lifestyle have a less diverse gut microbiome. So, what are you waiting for? Get moving using the exercise plans in Chapter Two.

Aim for 150 minutes of exercise each week! And I don't want to hear the old excuse that you're "just not an exercise person." There are so many different types of exercises out there that you can definitely find one you love. Do you like the water? Go swimming. Do you love to put your life in danger and feel the high of adrenaline rushing through your body? Go rock climbing. Do you love to challenge other people? Try fencing or boxing.

As we've already touched on, exercise improves gut motility, making waste leave your body quickly, so that harmful bacteria are not stuck up there just having a wild party at your expense!

5. KEEP AWAY THE SWEET POISON

Alcohol and sugar: These two jerks are so bad for human health; it's almost a cruel sick joke. Not only do they work hard to make you become addicted to your first taste, but they also feed all your harmful gut bacteria, so that the evil enemies in your Gut Kingdom can stage a coup.

Except for the odd glass of red wine here and there, you should also seriously consider cutting out alcohol from your diet if you want to be a gut-healthy hottie. The amount of bloating, weight gain, constipation, and diarrhea it causes is enough to make you look and feel ill.

Additionally, if you are craving sugar, turn to Mother Nature. The sugars she adds to fruits are OK for our gut health, in moderation, because of the amount of fiber and nutrients she also adds to offset their high sugar levels. When purchasing any food that is not in its natural state, read the ingredients because sugar is added to so much food these days - even in foods you'd never suspect, like tomato paste. The audacity!

6. TEA TIME!

No, we're not talking about sweet tea! Put the sugar jar back! We're talking about herbal teas - many of which taste far from sweet. In general, most herbal teas, like peppermint, cinnamon, ginger, and chamomile, are wonderful for treating digestive symptoms. Peppermint tea, for example, allows the muscles in your gastrointestinal tract to relax, preventing inflammation of your gut. A relaxed, gastrointestinal tract also stops bad microbiomes from reproducing. Don't forget to drink 2 cups of green tea daily, to reap all of its wonderful benefits, including healthy aging and a healthy gut.

7. LET'S DECAFFEINATE!

Have you ever wondered how the world was run before coffee became widespread? I would imagine we all slept more, had fewer eye bags, fewer jitters, and had better gut health. Although that may have been a disadvantage if the villager entrusted to stay awake overnight to watch out for wild animals accidentally fell asleep. Whoops! A hungry lion just showed up! And he thinks humans are great probiotics!

Caffeine shortens our sleep, which leads to more stress, leading to an unhealthy gut, and quick aging. If you absolutely must use caffeine, try drinks with smaller doses, like green tea or black tea. You should also be aware that decaffeinated coffee still contains some small amounts of caffeine in it that, over time, can also build up in your system and cause bad sleep patterns.

8. PROBIOTICS ARE YOUR NEW BFF

That's certainly what the lion in the story above thought. If a lion can take his probiotic intake seriously, why can't you? Eat more probiotic-rich foods and consider adding a daily probiotic supplement to your diet. By doing so, you are sending reinforcements with big guns and huge forearms to the probiotics already in your gut, so that they can win this war against the tyranny of your harmful gut pathogens.

9. FILL UP ON FRUITS AND FIBER

Fruit is the fastest digesting food, so eat fruits an hour before or after a meal. This aids digestion. They digest very well with leafy green vegetables. Contrariwise, avoid eating fruits with foods that digest slowly, such as proteins and starches. This can lead to bloating, indigestion, and flatulence. Fiber makes you regular, it prevents diarrhea and constipation, and it reduces any pain while "powdering your nose in the little girl's room"!

10. CHEW LIKE A SLOTH

Chew your food slowly, so that it can break down really well. This makes it much easier for the rest of your digestive system to do its work. Chewing like a sloth also helps you feel fuller, making you eat less between meals. Lastly, chewing slowly releases saliva, which tells your upper stomach muscles to relax, they are about to start work digesting! It also releases more stomach acid, enabling digestion.

11. FERMENTED FOODS ARE FUN

Fermented foods improve your gut diversity microbiome, which, as we all know, aids digestion. Eating foods such as yogurt, fermented cottage cheese, kimchi, kefir, and kombucha promotes conditions in your gut that healthy microbiota just love. They tell their friends about this great new place they just moved to, and their friends tell their friends, and before you know it, you have a whole gut-busting colony with a diverse group of microbiota.

12. LESS STRESS IS ALWAYS BEST

That rhymes! All right! And don't even try to act as though you don't find rhymes delightful and whimsical! How shmimsical! Stress causes inflammation in your body and has a negative impact on your immune system. These two things weaken your healthy bacteria, which, as you know, causes your evil bacteria to grow stronger and multiply. That's why less stress is the best, as this is the ideal condition for your healthy bacteria to thrive.

13. APPLE CIDER VINEGAR FOR THE WIN!

Apple cider vinegar (ACV) is just apple juice that has been fermented twice. Unfiltered apple cider vinegar contains enzymes, proteins, and bacteria that your gut just loves. In addition, it stimulates the production of stomach acid, helping to improve digestion. I can vouch for apple cider vinegar's effectiveness in keeping the stomach flat! That's how great for digestion it is.

Avoid filtered apple cider vinegar because it does not contain the enzymes, proteins, and bacteria that feed your gut. Add two tablespoons of ACV per glass of water, and try to drink it through a straw because it can wear out your enamel after a while. If you don't like the taste, try apple cider vinegar capsules.

14. THE BONE BROTH SECRET

Bone broth is made by slowly boiling animal bones and connective tissue. This helps you release the nutrient-rich gelatin inside the bone. The gelatin is packed full of glutamine, a very important nutrient for digestion. It also contains potassium, glucosamine, magnesium, proline, and glycine, which are amazing nutrients for your gut! Avoid store-bought bone broth as they tend to contain heavy metals.

15. MINDFULNESS MATTERS

Mindfulness involves bringing full awareness to your inner state: how you feel, the things that bother you, your innermost thoughts, etc. It is a way of checking in with yourself to clear all the unhealthy thoughts and emotions inside you and to find peace and calmness regardless of what is going on in your personal life.

Mindfulness is a great way of relieving stress, anxiety, and other negative emotions. It involves using gratitude, acceptance, and forgiveness to boost your mental and emotional health. As we will discuss in the next chapter, your mental health is just as important for improving your gut health as your physical health is.

If you find mindfulness on its own boring, try adding yoga, Pilates, or other forms of exercises to your practice.

PART III

RECHARGE YOUR MIND & BODY

7

ENS: THE GUT-BRAIN CONNECTION

> *"Your gut is your second brain."*
>
> — DR. MICHAEL GERSHON

Did you know that your gut is known as your body's second brain? It's quite fascinating! I don't want to ruin it for you, so let's just dig right in! All I'll do is give you a little teaser by telling you all the juicy topics this chapter will discuss: notably, our gut-brain connection, and how you can utilize that to benefit your mental health and/or cognitive functions. The Enteric nervous system, the gut-brain axis, and the role gut health plays in your mental health.

This summer... Get ready for the explosive gut-brain event of the century,,, in this chapter! Starring, your sexy gut ... in a red bikini! Your brain, draped in pink and coming off of a stint in sugar-high rehab! Your nervous system! And, guest starring, Digesty-Award winner, YOU in a figure-hugging, abs-popping, jaw-dropping gown! It's the most explosive event of the century!!

THE GUT-BRAIN AXIS: A BENEFICIAL RELATIONSHIP

Although it's not as complex a computer as our regular brains, the enteric nervous system, which regulates our guts, uses the same chemicals and cells as that of our brain, except it uses it to help us digest our food and to inform the brain when something is wrong. In short, your gut and brain work together, constantly communicating with each other to keep you healthy. This is why when you are in danger, you feel that sense of danger in your gut, even before your brain can begin flashing warning signs. It's also why bad news seems to hit us in our guts instead of our brains. The phrase, "My gut was right," suddenly makes a lot of scientific sense.

Braden Kuo, co-executive director of the Center for Neurointestinal Health at

Massachusetts General Hospital (MGH) and assistant professor of medicine at Harvard Medical School says:

"There is immense crosstalk between these two large nerve centers. This crosstalk affects how we feel and perceive gastrointestinal (GI) symptoms and impacts our quality of life."

Your gut and brain are constantly communicating with each other. That's why, when you are anxious and stressed, you may begin to experience butterflies before a big date with that hunk you've been eyeing, or have abdominal pain, nausea, or diarrhea, when you feel severely stressed or anxious. If you also find that you cannot watch a cooking show without suddenly having the desire to eat, that's because your brain sees something that looks good, so it communicates with your gut to get ready for food. This is kind of weird because you would think that with how sophisticated our brain is, it would have learned how to distinguish between pixelated food and real food by now. Silly brain!

So, if you really think about it, an unhealthy gut is like having an unhealthy brain. It's pretty much like making yourself disabled for absolutely no reason whatsoever. Since the bacteria in your gut affects your mood, behavior, and your cognition, then it is abundantly clear that you have to take your gut health seriously to have good mental health. In fact, many doctors now treat gastrointestinal disorders with cognitive approaches that you would think only belong in a psychiatrist's office, such as talk therapy, relaxation therapy, and hypnosis.

Many recent research studies now show categorically that gut health affects our brain, and brain health affects our gut. One recent study found that people who work high-stress jobs, such as "fire and ambulance services, police departments, hospitals, and defense forces... in complex, taxing and stressful environments," can improve their cognitive performance when they take their gut health seriously. In fact, scientists have recently discovered that people with Alzheimer's disease. A chronic condition that deteriorates brain function, "has a unique, and less diverse, community of gut microorganisms than their healthy counterparts," suffering especially from a decrease in the bacteria, Bifidobacterium.

Scientists are still at the beginning of their understanding of this deep interconnection between our gut health and our brain health. Dr. William Depaolo, a UW (University of Washington) Medicine gastroenterologist and director of the UW Center for Microbiome Sciences & Therapeutics said: "The role of the microbiome in health and disease is an exciting area at the forefront of science, but the field is in its infancy. I think about the microbiome like a biologist thinks about the deep sea. We know there's something down there, and we finally have the technology to help us see who's actually there and how they are influencing our bodies and brains".

The two are basically like Cinderella's step-sisters, working closely together, except, in this case, they are working together for your general health, not to be jerks to Cinderella. In fact, your gut contains hundreds of millions of neurons, all of which are connected to your brain through the nervous system. I wonder how all those wires are kept neat! The biggest nerve connecting Cinderella's step-sisters is a nerve known as the vagus nerve. Indeed, people who have a vagus nerve that doesn't work as best as it should tend to suffer from digestive disorders, such as IBS.

By now, you see how this all works. Basically, the gut-brain axis is incredibly connected and far more important for our health than scientists formerly thought. Did I mention that they're interconnected? I think I forgot to mention that! Plus, as we already discussed previously, your gut and brain both produce hormones, so, in this way, they work side-by-side to achieve equilibrium in your body.

THE ENTERIC NERVOUS SYSTEM: A TWO-WAY STREET

The enteric nervous system (ENS) is the bad boy of your gut. Dr. Jay Pasricha,

M.D., director of the Johns Hopkins Center for Neurogastroenterology, describes it as incapable of thought "as we know it" but still responsible for "controlling digestion, from swallowing to the release of enzymes that break down food to the control of blood flow that helps with nutrient absorption to elimination."

So what exactly is your ENS? Well, it is an extensive system of neurons that pretty much work independently according to their own rules. They wear slick black leather jackets, take whatever they want and do whatever they want. To be fair, they do work in tandem with the central nervous system, including your brain, but they are the only part of your digestive system that can work on their own without communicating with your brain. Just real bad boys!

The ENS is a 30-feet-or-so-long pathway located in the esophagus, stomach, small intestine, large intestine and rectum. It pretty much stretches through your entire gastrointestinal tract. It contains between 200 - 600 million neurons in charge of carrying messages from your central nervous system to your other organs. You know how we've mentioned peristalsis a few times in this book? Well, guess which bad boy is in charge of it? The ENS, despite being a bad boy, it also acts as a sort of a cop or snitch. It reacts to the food you've eaten, then tells on you to your CNS. So, if you ate that triple chocolate fudge caramel cookie, then, first of all, shame on you! Second of all, share the recipe! Third of all, your ENS has snitched to your central nervous system. While snitches do get stitches, it is important to note that this snitching is for your own good because knowing what you ate is very important if your body is to react properly to it. You certainly don't want to eat something incredibly sweet and decadent and then not have your CNS know about it. How else would it know to trigger the release of insulin? And what if you eat something that gives you food poisoning? Guess what triggers the vomit and diarrhea response to eject the bad bacteria or virus? You guessed it! So, in this case, snitches do not get stitches. They get accolades!

The ENS is also constantly alert to watch out for instances when you change your diet. Why? Well, digesting that triple chocolate fudge caramel cookie is going to be a lot easier than digesting some brown rice with peas and falafel patties. So, your ENS needs to keep up with changing digestion needs in your digestive tract. Sometimes these digestive changes might even come in the form of being infected with an outside pathogen, like a virus or bacteria that infects your gastrointestinal tract and makes you ill.

Furthermore, your gut microbiota has an effect on the ENS, so keeping a healthy gut will also improve your ENS's strength, efficacy, and general bad boy-ness. Your ENS is in charge of very important functions in your body, like blood flow, hormone release, motility (peristalsis), and secretions. In that way, it is slightly similar to the central nervous system, which controls various parts of your digestive system too, including voluntary bowel movements and stomach secretions.

Do your best to take care of your ENS by cultivating a healthy microflora. Since it is so paramount to your digestive health, an unhealthy ENS can lead to digestive issues when its neurons are disrupted or injured. This, in turn, can lead to digestive issues.

THE GUT AFFECTS THE BRAIN ... AND VICE-VERSA

In recent years, scientists are uncovering how our gut microflora actually keeps our brain healthy and even shapes our thoughts and behaviors. How odd!

This is still a pioneering new field that needs a lot of research, but scientists believe that our gut microbes may communicate with our brains through numerous pathways, including the vagus nerve. Just as we've seen a link between Alzheimer's and gut dysbiosis, scientists also think that the bacteria, Lactobacillus rhamnosus JB1 improves mood when you're feeling anxious or depressed. Dr. John Cryan, a professor of anatomy and neuroscience at University College Cork explains, "In medicine, we tend to compartmentalize the body, so, when we talk about issues with the brain, we tend to think about the neck upwards. But we need to frame things evolutionarily. It's important to remember that microbes were here before humans existed, so we have evolved with these 'friends with benefits.' There has never been a time when the brain existed without the signals coming from the microbes. What if these signals are actually really important in determining how we feel, how we behave, and how we respond? And could we modulate these microbes therapeutically to improve thinking, behavior, and brain health?"

So far, most of the research on the link between gut health and the brain has been done on mice because it is such a new field in the understanding of gut health. What we do know, however, is that a healthy gut provides a much better likelihood of developing a healthy brain.

GUT HEALTH & MENTAL HEALTH

When it comes to neurodegenerative disease and mood disorders, the ENS is an important player. Although there is still a lot of research to be done, scientists believe that a disordered (unhealthy) ENS can cause anxiety, depression, multiple sclerosis, SAD (social anxiety disorder), Parkinson's disease, Alzheimer's, and OCD (Obsessive Compulsive Disorder). The ENS keeps our gut health in balance (homeostasis). If it is not healthy, this can lead to severe imbalances that could threaten your mental health.

LET'S TALK LIFESTYLE

Your gut is called your second brain for a reason: because it is. This gut-brain connection is fascinating and gives us a really good clue into how our bodies work. One thing research duplicates is that people with a healthy gut have better mental health and cognitive functions. That means that they are able to think better, plan better, strategize better, and so on. We also now know that a healthy gut-brain connection improves your mental health and reduces the chances of your brain health deteriorating as you age.

To optimize your mental health, follow the following gut health tips:

- Ensure you are doing activities such as yoga to reduce stress and improve the health of your microflora.
- Try to stick to a regular sleep pattern in a comfortable environment. This will help ensure you get good quality sleep on a regular basis.
- Use gardening and raise plants around the house to naturally lower your stress levels.
- Reduce your caffeine intake. Over time, caffeine can cause insomnia, making you even more stressed and leading to anxiety.
- Eat foods rich in B vitamins. B vitamins reduce your risk of depression.
- Spend time with those you love. This causes your body to release stress-busting hormones, keeping your microflora in a healthy state.

There you have it! One of the keys to good mental health is to eat healthily. Do you want to improve your thinking, act well, be fully alert in your day-to-day life, prevent mental health disorders, and just be a classy, well-rounded hottie? Eat for your gut health! It's a positive cycle really. When you eat well, your physical health improves, which gives you the energy to also prioritize your mental health. Good mental health, in turn, then gives you the motivation to take care of your physical health. And on and on it goes until you achieve ultimate health and transcend health levels previously unknown to mankind.

8

MODULATED: MANAGING YOUR MOOD WITH FOOD

> *"Laughter is brightest where food is best."*
>
> — IRISH PROVERB

It's not just your mental health that is influenced by those tiny micro-organisms living in your car. It's also your mood. In the final chapter of this book, we will explore how food can actually manage your mood and regulate your emotions.

If you've ever wondered why sometimes you feel hangry (hungry + angry), all the science behind things, like sugar highs (feeling really amazing when you eat something with a lot of sugar), sugar crashes (when you spike your insulin through sugary snacks then suddenly have a drop in energy), and food commas (that

Thanksgiving feeling when you eat so much that you feel tired and sluggish afterward), then you're in luck. Here is where we'll examine how our guts play a role in these moods and emotions. Lastly, this chapter will end with a cheat sheet for you to refer to whenever you feel as though your emotions are unmanageable.

ARE YOU REALLY "HANGRY"?

I like to be a respectful person. I believe that everyone should be treated with respect and dignity. I say, "Thank you," and I say, "Please." I apologize when I'm wrong, and I try to be kind and patient with people, even when they may not be on their best behavior. But, despite these values of compassion, empathy, human dignity, and kindness being drilled into me from a young age, I am challenged the minute my blood sugar gets low. Sometimes, I don't notice until, out of the blue, I get snappy, turn into a deranged monster, and raise a loud dinosaur shriek at whoever is nearby. It took me a while to notice this pattern but, now, whenever my usually-pleasant self turns into the monster you imagined lived under your bed as a child, I know it's time to reach for a healthy snack. This is what is known as being "hangry."

We get hangry because our brains need glucose to function properly. If you remember your Biology lessons at school, you were taught that carbohydrates break down into glucose (simple sugars), proteins break down into amino acids, and fats break down into free fatty acids. These macronutrients then pass through your entire body, through your blood, so that your organs and tissues can slurp up what they need. Of course, after a while, your organs and tissues have slurped up all the nutrients in your blood, which is around the time your body starts to tell you that you need to eat again. For most people, that's pretty OK. We can wait another hour or two before we get some more nutrients in. It's just that our brain is a bit diva-ish. It needs glucose NOW! If it does not get glucose NOW, it goes on strike. It literally just decides to stop doing its job properly until you come to your senses, recognize who the boss is around here and provide some damn glucose. Let's just say the brain turns things around here, and you better recognize!

You suddenly start to act in very socially unacceptable ways. Just like me, you probably get a bit snappy at people when your glucose is low. You find it difficult to concentrate, you start to make silly mistakes, you can't even speak properly, you're grumpy ... it's just a mess. Here is how Dr. Veronica Santini, a clinical assistant professor, of neurology and neurological sciences at Stanford Health Care explains it, "The part of our brains associated with hunger, fear, anxiety, and anger is called the limbic system. It starts automatic responses we have before they even come to consciousness in the higher brain area, which takes information from the limbic system and the environment and then modulates these primitive responses. This is why we're not walking around yelling at everybody. But if you have low glucose levels, it means higher brain functions are not working as well as they could be, so there may be a breakdown in those higher brain functions that help us modulate primitive responses." Or, in more simplistic terms, we act like classless Neanderthals when we are hangry. I know I certainly do.

HERE'S WHY YOU CALM DOWN ONCE YOU'VE EATEN SOMETHING

Once you've eaten something, your brain calls off the strike. It's asserted dominance and reminded you who's in charge, and it hopes you've learned your lesson about depriving it of glucose. Well, that and the fact that the hormone ghrelin lowers. Ghrelin is the hunger hormone. It resides in your stomach. When your stomach is empty, the hormone level shoots up, which sends bright warning signals to your brain that it needs to go on strike. When you eat, the hormone level goes down, and your brain calls off the strike. It's also why sometimes you eat, and you still want to eat more. You have not eaten enough (especially enough carbohydrates), so the ghrelin level is still high enough for your brain to give you sass. That's why some carbohydrates and proteins, such as rice and eggs, are so satiating. They fill you up, causing ghrelin levels to lower significantly.

Not only does ghrelin moderate your appetite, increasing it when you are hungry and decreasing it when you are full, but it also makes you take in plenty of calories and fat. You see, this hormone was trained on the job during a time when humans did not have consistent meals. So it learned to keep humans alive by storing fat and encouraging you to eat a lot. Well, now, when you can order extra meat lovers pizza if you want, ghrelin has not adapted to the new way of life and just wants to keep you full and satiated at all times. Hence, when you eat and you are full, your brain rewards you with the feel-good hormone, dopamine, so you keep eating. Those two jerks are in on this together! The audacity to dare try to keep you alive! Well, of course, once ghrelin levels decrease and mood-boosting dopamine and serotonin levels increase, you feel so good, the anger just dissipates.

A similar mechanism occurs when you are constantly in a state of stress. Your adrenal glands release the hormone cortisol to help you deal with the stress.

Cortisol naturally increases your appetite and generally increases people's motivation, which includes your motivation to eat. This, of course, then makes it difficult to lose weight and to lose body fat. Again, those jerks!

USING FOOD TO MANAGE MOOD

Basically, it's not just what we do that affects our mood. Alas! It's also when we eat and how we eat. Remember when we talked about hormones constantly working to keep all the processes within our bodies working efficiently, and to keep us healthy? Well, you can see now how these hormones are actually constantly working, reacting to everything that you do to your body, put in your body and even reacting to each other, to the different processes going on in different parts of your body.

The great news is that you don't really have to learn too much at this stage in the book because all the advice given in chapters before this also works to keep your hormones in a stable state so that you are always constantly managing your mood without trying too hard. For instance, if you exercise often, as we discussed in Chapter Two, you will naturally eat more regularly because your metabolism will be boosted. Eating more regularly means that your glucose levels do not suddenly drop, also meaning that your brain doesn't go on strike and you don't get hangry. One final piece of advice I would give is to always have healthy snacks in your office, at home, in your car, in your lover's apartment, and so on. That way, when hunger strikes (no pun intended) you can placate your brain as quickly as possible, so it doesn't go on strike!

Personally, no matter how much I eat the night before, I am always hungry the next morning. That's why I always ensure to bake and freeze healthy breakfast muffins. That way I have something to eat with my morning green tea, to power me through my morning routine. I don't say this so that you'll copy me. More so that you recognize that different habits and patterns work for everyone. The more you get stuck in a healthy living lifestyle, the more you'll figure out what works for you.

EAT THIS, NOT THAT

Use this food cheat sheet as a way to manage your moods and emotions. The nutrients in each food listed help alleviate common negative emotions. It's kind of like how illicit drugs make the negative emotions go away but, instead of drugs, you use food since it's way healthier, definitely cheaper, and you don't have to do jail time if you're caught buying it. Plus, you don't need a "guy" to buy these foods. Just go to your local food dealer, also known as a "supermarket."

Food Mood Cheat Sheet

Sadness

- Fruits and vegetables
- Tofu
- Milk
- Fish and seafood
- Beans
- Wholegrains
- Nuts
- Dark, green leafy vegetables
- Flaxseed oil
- Canola oil
- Lean meats
- Lean proteins

Low (lethargic, upset, etc.)

- Poultry (without the skin)
- Seafood, especially fish
- Lean meat
- Plenty of water
- Citrus fruits

- Berries
- Melons
- Dark, green leafy vegetables

Tired/Fatigue

- Watermelon
- Kale
- Spinach
- Bee pollen
- Dates
- Chia seeds
- Bananas
- Almonds
- Avocados
- Eggs

Restless/Anxious

- Dark, green leafy vegetables
- Cashews
- Oysters
- Turkey breast
- Chamomile tea
- Oatmeal
- Green tea
- Eggs

- Yogurt
- Beets
- Blueberries
- Milk
- Dark chocolate
- Turmeric
- Seeds
- Pistachios
- Oranges
- Seaweed
- Salmon

Dazed (Brain Fog)

- Olive oil
- Salmon
- Avocados
- Dark, green leafy vegetables

Boosting happiness

- Fatty fish
- Fermented foods
- Bananas
- Nuts
- Seeds
- Oatmeal\Dark chocolate

- Berries
- Beans
- Lentils

Stressed

- Artichokes
- Tahini
- Parsley
- Garlic
- Chamomile tea
- Sweet potatoes
- Fatty fish
- Organ meats
- Chickpeas
- Matcha powder
- Swiss chard
- Eggs
- Sunflower seeds
- Acerola cherry powder
- Broccoli
- Blueberries

CONCLUSION

By now, you're probably rearing to go. Many of my clients are often shocked how easy it is to achieve a new life, bursting with energy and better health. All I needed to do was change my diet? Why didn't anyone tell me how easy it was? I have heard this phrase over and over again, that I now come to expect it.

If you really think about it, it's quite surprising how no one teaches us the importance of gut health at school. I have a feeling that governments would spend a lot less on healthcare if the absolute importance of gut health was drilled into us as children. I know I sure would have made better health choices as a child and a young adult. What's even stranger is that my school would offer the most unhealthy food ever to us kids. Sure, they tried to change it up a bit towards the end of my time there, but the healthy versions were so gross, of course, none of us ate it, and they used it as an excuse to continue feeding us cheap-to-buy and equally cheap-to-prepare "food." I use the word "food" here very loosely.

If I had known the wide variety of chronic illnesses, I could at least have taken preventative steps to avoid them by eating well. Then I certainly would have replaced chocolate for apples once in a while. I would have bought more fruits and vegetables, more whole grains, and more legumes. Still, we cannot change the past. I did not know then, but I know now, so I do better. And the same applies to you. You cannot change what you've eaten, but you certainly can start now towards healing gut dysbiosis, feeding your good guy gut bacteria, and bringing in a new reign of good microbiota in your gut. The evil microflora shall be banished from your gut kingdom, and peace shall reign supreme in all the land! It's science!

As a practitioner of a gut-healthy diet myself, I have to admit that I love this diet because it enables me to feel better and look better whilst still eating delicious food and living a full, happy life. Who doesn't want that? Who doesn't want to try on a dress without worrying that you would look like you are smuggling watermelons around your stomach area? Who wouldn't want to wake up feeling energized and not needing to worry about falling ill all the time because your immune system has gone into hyper overdrive? Who doesn't love the ladylike convenience of a smooth, pain-free, hassle-free bowel movement that even the gods themselves would kill for? And who certainly doesn't enjoy living life burp-free and free of any other gases trapped inside you that might seek escape from their confinement?

We all want to live healthy, happy lives devoid of any gastrointestinal embarrassments or accidents. In this book, I have taught you how to do just that, providing you with all the information you need to be a gut health hottie. You now know what your microbiome is and why hotties like you and I don't even DO gut dysbiosis! We're just too classy for all that! Now you know how to optimize your digestion, how to create a flat tummy with my handy diet plan, and how to help your flat tummy along using my exercise plans. You have the tools you need to restore your estrobolome, destroy hormonal imbalance, and eat for healthy aging. Lastly, you can improve your mental health, cognition, and mood anytime you want by following the advice on your gut-brain connection and managing your mood.

Et voila! A gut health hottie is born! Out of the clay, you are reborn, remolded, beautiful, healthy, stunning! The gods themselves gasp in awe! They have never seen a human with such a healthy microflora! How does she do it? What is her secret?

Well, the secret is this book! Now that you know how important gut health is, you're equipped to make better, more informed decisions about your health, body, and mind. You are now more aware - and therefore can be more cautious - about the long-term effects that your food, exercise, and lifestyle choices can have on your overall health.

Today, scientists are not moving slowly towards thinking of our gut microbiome not just as a group of bacteria living together but as an organ in its own right. That's how important these organisms are to your entire life. Take care of them and they will take care of you.

Now that you are well on your way to becoming your own version of a gut-healthy hottie, you are in a perfect position to help someone else. By simply leaving your honest opinion on Amazon, you will help other women like yourself find the support they are looking for and help start them on their own journey to feeling and looking great.

ANOTHER GIFT TO MY READERS...

Please enjoy these downloadable PDFs of the

10, 30, 60 Exercise Program

&

30-Day Flat Tummy Meal Plan

Scan the QR Codes below!

10,30,60 Exercise Program

30-Day Flat Tummy Meal Plan

BIBLIOGRAPHY

"10 Effects of Stress on Your Face, and How to Lower Anxiety." 2020. Healthline. June 25, 2020. https://www.healthline.com/health/stress-on-face#takeaway.

"15 Mood-Boosting Foods." 2011. Prevention. November 3, 2011. https://www.prevention.com/health/a20462615/food-and-mood-the-best-foo ds-to-make-you-feel-better/.

"18 of the Best Stress-Relieving Foods." 2020. Healthline. June 8, 2020. https://www.healthline.com/nutrition/stress-relieving-foods#15.-Broccoli.

"2-Ingredient (More or Less) Sweet Potato Pancakes." 2023. Cooking Light. Accessed April 24, 2023. https://www.cookinglight.com/recipes/2-ingredient-sweet-potato-pancakes.

"20 Powerful Journal Prompts for Stress Relief." 2020. Through the Phases. April 24, 2020. https://www.throughthephases.com/jour nal-prompts-for-stress-relief/.

"4 Easy Stretches to Speed up Digestion." 2015. Good Housekeeping. December 16, 2015. https://www.goodhousekeeping.-com/uk/health/healthy-eating/a558368/easystretches-that-help-digestion/.

"4 Nutritionist-Approved Foods to Boost Your Brain and Fight Fatig." 2018. Healthline. October 26, 2018. https://www.healthline.com/health/food-nutrition/brain-food-for-fatigue.

7 Surprising Ways Your Gut Health Affects Your Fitness." 2023. Hyperbiotics. Accessed April 11, 2023. https://www.hyperbiotics.-com/blogs/recent-articles/7-surprising-ways-your-g ut-health-affects-your-fitness.

Ackerman, Courtney. 2019. "83 Benefits of Journaling for Depression, Anxiety, and Stress." PositivePsychology.com. July 10, 2019. https://positivepsychology.com/benefits-of-journaling/.

"Age Gracefully with These 12 Stress Relief Tips | MaxLiving." 2020. June 1, 2020. https://maxliving.com/healthy-articles/stress-relief-tips-to-age-gracefully/.

Alyssa. 2022. "Detox Turmeric Lentil Soup (Easy Detox Vegetable Soup Recipe!)." Simply Quinoa. May 11, 2022.

https://www.simplyquinoa.com/detox-turmeric-lentil-soup/.

"Are Telomeres the Key to Aging and Cancer." 2012. Utah.edu. 2012. https://learn.genetics.utah.edu/content/basics/telomeres/.

Baier, Anne DeLotto. 2021. "USF Health Researcher Studies Gut Microbiome to Improve Brain Health, Decrease Age-Related Diseases." USF Health News. September 3, 2021. https://hscweb3.hsc.usf.edu/blog/2021/09/03/usf-health-researcher-studies-gut-microbiome-to-improve-brain-health-decrease-age-related-diseases/.

"Berry-Kefir Smoothie." 2023. EatingWell. https://www.eatingwell.com/recipe/257793/berry-kefir-smoothie/.

"Berry Overnight Oats." 2023. Allrecipes. https://www.allrecipes.com/recipe/257039/berry-overnight-oats/.

"Best Stretches for Tight Hamstrings: 8 Methods." 2022. Www.medicalnewstoday.com. June 24, 2022. https://www.medicalnewstoday.com/articles/323703#best-stretches.

Brazil, London. 2023. "Peanut Butter Banana Overnight Oats." Evolving Table. January 10, 2023. https://www.evolvingtable.com/peanut-butter-banana-overnight-oats/.

"Breaking down the Estrobolome with Moira Bradfield | FX Medicine." 2021. Www.fxmedicine.com.au. https://www.fxmedicine.com.au/podcast/breaking-down-estrobolome-moirabradfield.

"Can You Exercise with Digestive Problems?" 2023. MedicineNet. https://www.medicinenet.com/can_you_exercise_with_digestive_problems/a rticle.htm.

"Chronological vs. Biological Aging: Differences & More." 2023. Healthline. https://www.healthline.com/health/chronological-ageing#healthy-aging.

Cleveland Clinic. 2013. "Estrogen and Cancer: Information & Risks |

Cleveland Clinic." Cleveland Clinic. 2013. https://my.clevelandclinic.org/health/diseases/10312-estrogen-dependent-can cers.

Cleveland Clinic. 2022. "Hormonal Imbalance: Causes, Symptoms & Treatment." Cleveland Clinic. April 4, 2022. https://my.cleveland clinic.org/health/diseases/22673-hormonal-imbalance.

ckgdmchange. 2022. "Top 10 Daily Habits to Promote Hormone Balance." Nutrition 4 Change. March 22, 2022. https://nutrition4change.com/articles/top-10-daily-habits-to-promote-hormo ne-balance/.

"Comforting Slow Cooker Vegetable Stew with Only 10 Minutes Prep." 2023. The Spruce Eats. Accessed May 2, 2023. https://www.thes pruceeats.com/slow-cooker-vegetable-stew-2246305.

"Common Digestive Disorders: Symptoms and Treatments." 2021. Www.medicalnewstoday.com. September 10, 2021. https://www.medicalnewstoday.com/articles/list-of-digestive-disorders#celiac -disease.

Costa, M. 2000. "Anatomy and Physiology of the Enteric Nervous System." Gut 47 (90004): 15iv19. https://doi.org/10.1136/gut.47. suppl_4.iv15.

Dalthorp, R. 2023. "Hormone Balancing Diet." Balance Women's Health. https://balancewomenshealth.com/wp-content/uploads/2020/03/Hormone_ Balance_Diet.pdf.

Dawnie2u. 2023. "Thai Carrot Soup Recipe - Food.com." Food. 2023. https://www.food.com/recipe/thai-carrot-soup-191957.

De Filippo, Carlotta, Monica Di Paola, Matteo Ramazzotti, Davide Albanese, Giuseppe Pieraccini, Elena Banci, Franco Miglietta, Duccio Cavalieri, and Paolo Lionetti. 2017. "Diet, Environments, and Gut Microbiota. A Preliminary Investigation in Children Living in Rural and Urban Burkina Faso and Italy." Frontiers in Microbiology 8 (October). https://doi.org/10.3389/fmicb.2017. 01979.

"Depression & Diet: 6 Foods That Fight Depression." 2012. Healthline. March 26, 2012. https://www.healthline.com/health/depression/ diet#Foods-that-Might-Help.

"Diet and Gastrointestinal Disease: 8 Best Foods for Gut Health." 2023.

Www.nebraskamed.com. https://www.nebraskamed.com/gastrointestinal-care/diet-and-gastrointestinal disease-8-best-foods-for-gut-health.

"Enteric Nervous System: Anatomy, Function, and Treatment." 2023. Verywell Health. https://www.verywellhealth.com/enteric-nervous-system-5112820.

"Estrobolome - the Gut-Hormone Connection." 2023. Dr. Karen Wallace, ND | Dartmouth, Nova Scotia. Accessed April 29, 2023. http://drkarenwallace.com/blog-drkaren-naturopathic-dartmouth/2020/1/23/ the-gut-estrogen-connection.

"Exercises to Improve Digestion." 2023. AXA Health. https://www.axahealth.co.uk/health-information/gut-health/exercises-to-impr ove-digestion/.

Ezhilarasan, Devaraj. 2020. "Critical Role of Estrogen in the Progression of Chronic Liver Diseases." Hepatobiliary & Pancreatic Diseases International 19 (5): 429–34. https://doi.org/10.1016/j.hbpd.2020.03.011.

"From Sleepy to Supercharged: 10 Foods for Morning Fatigue." 2018. Healthline. September 21, 2018. https://www.healthline.-com/health/food-nutrition/morning-fatigue#3.-Almon ds.

Funston, Lindsay, Christina Oehler Updated May 21, and 2020. "20 Foods That Can Help Relieve Stress." Health.com. https://www.health.com/food/stress-relieving-foods.

Galloway, Jordan. 2022. "3 Signs of a Healthy Gut from a Gastroenterologist." Well+Good. April 29, 2022. https://www.wellandgood.com/signs-healthy-gut/.

Gayle. 2016. "Honey Garlic Salmon and Quinoa Bowl." Pumpkin 'N Spice. September 1, 2016. https://www.pumpkinnspice.com/honey-garlic-salmon-quinoa-bowl/.

"Gentle Exercises to Help Digestion: Yoga, Tai Chi, and More." 2019. Healthline. March 6, 2019. https://www.healthline.com/health/epi/exercises-digestion#takeaway.

"Ghrelin: The 'Hunger Hormone' Explained." 2016. Healthline. June 24, 2016. https://www.healthline.com/nutrition/ghrelin#TOC_TITLE_HDR_5.

Gina. 2020. "Healthy Cod Fish Tacos (Quick and Easy Recipe)." Skinnytaste. February 28, 2020. https://www.skinnytaste.com/cod-fish-tacos/.

"Greek Kale Salad with Quinoa & Chicken." 2023. EatingWell. https://www.eatingwell.com/recipe/262450/greek-kale-salad-with-quinoa-chi cken/.

"Green Salad with Edamame & Beets." 2023. EatingWell. https://www.eatingwell.com/recipe/259814/green-salad-with-edamame-beets/.

GIS. 2018. "Physical Activity and GI Health." Gastrointestinal Society. 2018. https://badgut.org/information-centre/a-z-digestive-topics/physical-activity-a nd-gi-health/.

Gupta, Ekta. 2021. "GERD Diet: Foods That Help with Acid Reflux (Heartburn)." Www.hopkinsmedicine.org. 2021. https://www.hopkinsmedicine.org/health/wellness-and-prevention/gerd-diet-f oods-that-help-with-acid-reflux-heartburn.

"Gut Health and Hormones." 2023. Leigh Ann Scott MD, Las Colinas, Irving TX. https://www.leighannscottmd.com/additional-testing/gut-health-and-hormon es/.

Harvard Health Publishing. 2018. "Why Stress Causes People to Overeat." Harvard Health. Harvard Health. July 18, 2018. https://www.health.harvard.edu/staying-healthy/why-stress-causes-people-toovereat.

Head, Ally. 2022. "11 Simple Gut Health Hacks That Promise to Boost Your Wellbeing (plus Skin, Digestion, and More)." Marie Claire UK. January 18, 2022. https://www.marieclaire.co.uk/life/health-fitness/gut-health-hacks-762014.

"Healthy Avocado Chickpea Salad (10-Minute Recipe!)." 2021. Hint of Healthy. June 25, 2021. https://www.hintofhealthy.com/avocado-chickpea-salad/.

Hendley, Joyce, 2021. "How Food Can Help You Look and Feel More Youthful—Here's What the Science Says," April 15, 2021. https://www.eatingwell.com/article/7898812/how-food-can-help-you-look-an d-feel-more-youthful-heres-what-the-science-says/.

"Homemade Garlic Aioli {5 Mins Prep!}." 2020. Spend with Pennies. May 22, 2020. https://www.spendwithpennies.com/aioli/.

Honey, Dash of. 2023. "Buddha Bowl with Creamy Miso Sauce." Dash of Honey. January 1, 2023. https://dashofhoney.ca/en/buddha-bowl-with-creamy-miso-sauce/.

"Hormones & Gut Health: The Estrobolome & Hormone Balance." 2020. Marion Gluck. June 29, 2020. https://www.mariongluckclinic.com/blog/hormones-and-gut-health-the-estro bolome-and-hormone-balance.html.

"How Exercise Affects Your Digestion - Manhattan Gastroenterology." 2017. Manhattan Gastroenterology. July 18, 2017. https://www.manhattangastroenterology.com/exercise-affects-digestion/.

"How to Improve Gut Health: 16 Simple Hacks for Your Gut in 2020." 2019. Atlas Biomed Blog | Take Control of Your Health with No-Nonsense News on Lifestyle, Gut Microbes and Genetics. December 31, 2019. https://atlasbiomed.com/blog/16-easy-hacks-to-enhance-your-gut-health-ever y-day-in-2020/.

"How to Trick Yourself into Making Exercise a Habit." 2023. NBC News. https://www.nbcnews.com/better/health/6-mental-tricks-tricks-help-make-ex ercise-habit-ncna914386.

"How Your Gut Microbiome Influences Your Hormones." 2019. Bulletproof. June 6, 2019. https://www.bulletproof.com/gut-health/gut-microbiome-hormones/.

HQ, Healthy Smoothie. 2015. "Greek Yogurt Strawberry Smoothie." Healthy Smoothie HQ. January 15, 2015. https://www.healthys moothiehq.com/greek-yogurt-strawberry-smoothie.

"IBS Home Remedies That Work: Lifestyle and Diet Tips." 2017. Healthline. September 25, 2017. https://www.healthline.-com/health/ibs-home-remedies-that-work#_noHeade rPrefixed-Content.

"If Your Gut Health Is out of Whack, You Could Be Missing These Important Foods." 2022. Mindbodygreen. May 27, 2022. https://www.mindbodygreen.com/articles/gut-health-diet.

Islam, Sameer. 2021. "7 Natural Gut Health Hacks." Lubbock Gastroenterology. July 7, 2021. https://lubbockgastro.com/natural-gut-health-hacks/.

Joanne. 2022. "BEST Butternut Squash Soup Ever." Fifteen Spatulas. October 28, 2022. https://www.fifteenspatulas.com/butternut-squash-soup/.

Johns Hopkins Medicine. 2019. "The Brain-Gut Connection." John Hopkins Medicine. 2019.

https://www.hopkinsmedicine.org/health/wellness-and-prevention/the-braingut-connection.

Jones, Rebel. 2022. "79 Self Care Quotes for Your Mind, Body & Soul." Happier Human. June 21, 2022. https://www.happierhuman.com/self-care-quotes/.

Julia. (2020, March 6). Arugula Tomato Salad - Julia's Album. Julia's Album. https://juliasalbum.com/arugula-tomato-salad/

Lastowka, L. 2023. "Vegetarian Niçoise Salad." EatingWell. https://www.eatingwell.com/recipe/270570/vegetarian-nicoise-salad/.

"Low-FODMAP Tomato and Leek Frittata | Low FODMAP Diet by FODMAP Life." 2016. Www.fodmaplife.com. June 17, 2016. http://www.fodmaplife.com/2016/06/17/low-fodmap-tomato-and-leek-frittata

/.

Kerr, Courtney. 2021. "Top 50 Motivational Workout Quotes." Upper Hand. April 25, 2021. https://upperhand.com/50-motivational-workout-quotes/.

Larson, Lauren, MS, and RDN. 2014. "Protecting Your Telomeres with the Right Food - Food & Nutrition Magazine." Foodandnutrition.org. February 6, 2014. https://foodandnutrition.org/blogs/stone-soup/protecting-telomeres-right-foo d/.

"Lifestyle." 2023. Headsup. https://www.headsup.org.au/your-mental-health/taking-care-of-yourself-andstaying-well/lifestyle.

"List of Digestive Disorders: 10 Common and Rare Conditions." 2021. Www.medicalnewstoday.com. January 19, 2021. https://www.medicalnewstoday.com/articles/list-of-digestive-disorders.

Macey, Deryn. 2021. "White Bean Chili." Running on Real Food. January 22, 2021. https://runningonrealfood.com/white-bean-chili/.

Marttinen, Maija, Reeta Ala-Jaakkola, Arja Laitila, and Markus J. Lehtinen. 2020. "Gut Microbiota, Probiotics and Physical Performance in Athletes and Physically Active Individuals." Nutrients 12 (10): 2936. https://doi.org/10.3390/nu12102936.

Maser, Rachel. 2017. "Shrimp Fajitas with Avocado Are Super Quick and Packed with Flavor!" Clean Food Crush. May 17, 2017. https://cleanfoodcrush.com/fast-clean-eating-shrimp-fajitas/.

Mauvais-Jarvis, Franck, Deborah J. Clegg, and Andrea L. Hevener. 2013. "The Role of Estrogens in Control of Energy Balance and Glucose Homeostasis." Endocrine Reviews 34 (3): 309–38. https://doi.org/10.1210/er.2012-1055.

Mayo Clinic. 2018. "Celiac Disease - Diagnosis and Treatment - Mayo Clinic." Mayoclinic.org. 2018. https://www.mayoclinic.org/diseases-conditions/celiac-disease/diagnosis-trea tment/drc-20352225.

MD, Robert H. Shmerling. 2023. "Gut Health Quotes to Inspire and Motivate You on Your Health Journey." Harvard School of Public Health. April 8, 2023. https://chgeharvard.org/gut-health-quotes-to-inspire-and-motivate-you-on-yo ur-health-journey/.

Minimalist Baker. 2017. "Gingery Mango & Berry Smoothie." Minimalist Baker. August 29, 2017. https://minimalistbaker.com/gingery-mango-berry-smoothie/.

Monroe, Sasha. 2020. ""Nourishing Yourself in a Way That Helps You Blossom in the Direction You Want to Go Is Attainable…." #BOLD. November 2, 2020. https://medium.com/be-bold/nourishing-yourself-in-a-way-that-helps-you-blossom-in-the-direction-you-want-to-go-is-attainable-ab9b1cb519b9#:

"Mood Food: 9 Foods That Can Really Boost Your Spirits." 2020. Healthline. February 5, 2020. https://www.healthline.com/nutrition/mood-food#1.-Fatty-fish.

"Most Delicious Falafel Recipe (Fried or Baked)." 2019. Downshiftology. July 19, 2019. https://downshiftology.com/recipes/falafel/.

Nast, Condé. 2018. "How to Improve Your Gut Health in 6 Easy Steps." Vogue. April 6, 2018. https://www.vogue.com/article/gut-digestive-health-best-expert-tips-nutritiou s-life-diet-sleep-stress-exercise-cleanse.

Natasha. 2017. "Healthy Baked Salmon Tacos." Salt and Lavender. January 17 2017. https://www.saltandlavender.com/healthy-baked-salmon-tacos/.

National Institutes of Health. 2015. "NIH Human Microbiome Project Defines Normal Bacterial Makeup of the Body." National Institutes of Health (NIH). August 31, 2015. https://www.nih.gov/news-events/news-releases/nih-human-microbiome-proj ect-defines-normal-bacterial-makeup-body.

Olympic Channel Writer. 2021. "Michael Phelps' 10000 Calories Diet: What the American Swimmer Ate While Training for Beijing Olympics?" Olympics.com. International Olympic Committee. May 16, 2021. https://olympics.com/en/news/michael-phelps-10000-calories-diet-what-theamerican-swimmer-ate-while-training-.

"Open-Face Turkey Burgers and Sweet Potato Fries." 2023. BigOven.com. https://www.bigoven.com/recipe/open-face-turkey-burgers-and-sweet-potatofries/1565802.

"Oxidative Stress: Definition, Effects on the Body, and Prevention." 2023. Healthline. https://www.healthline.com/health/oxidative-stress#takeaway.

Palmer, C. and Gupta, S. 2022. "Good vs. Bad Bacteria: 5 Tips to Improve Gut Health." Good Rx Health. December 13, 2022. https://www.goodrx.com/well-being/gut-health/good-bad-bacteria-gut-health

"Peanut Butter-Banana Cinnamon Toast." 2023. EatingWell. https://www.eatingwell.com/recipe/261628/peanut-butter-banana-cinnamontoast/.

Pietrangelo, Ann. 2017. "Crohn's Disease: Why Do I Feel This Way?" Healthline. Healthline Media. March 15, 2017. https://www.healthline.com/health/crohns-disease/effects-of.

Purves, Dale, George J. Augustine, David Fitzpatrick, Lawrence C. Katz, Anthony-Samuel LaMantia, James O. McNamara, and S. Mark Williams. 2001. "The Enteric Nervous System."

Neuroscience. 2nd Edition. https://www.ncbi.nlm.nih.gov/books/NBK11097/.

"Relaxation Techniques to Manage IBS Symptoms - about IBS." 2023 https://aboutibs.org/treatment/psychological-treatments/relax-ation-technique s-for-ibs/.

"Roasted Veggie & Hummus Pita Pockets." 2023. EatingWell. https://www.eatingwell.com/recipe/261292/roasted-veggie-hummus-pita-poc kets/.

Robertson, Ruairi. 2016. "10 Ways to Improve Your Gut Bacteria, Based on Science." Healthline. Healthline Media. November 18, 2016. https://www.healthline.com/nutrition/improve-gut-bacteria.

Romm, Aviva. 2021. "The Estrobolome: The Fascinating Way Your Gut Impacts Your Estrogen Levels." Aviva Romm, MD. April 13, 2021. https://avivaromm.com/estrobolome/.

Ruder, Debra Bradley. (2017). "The Gut and the Brain." Harvard. https://hms.harvard.edu/news-events/publications-archive/brain/gut-brain

Salis, Amanda. 2015. "The Science of 'Hangry:' Why Some People Get Grumpy When They're Hungry." CNN. July 20, 2015. https://edi-tion.cnn.com/2015/07/20/health/science-behind-being-hangry/ind ex.html.

Sally. 2021. "Healthy Whole Wheat Banana Walnut Muffins." Sally's Baking Addiction. August 26, 2021. https://sallysbakingaddiction.-com/whole-wheat-banana-nut-muffins/#tasty-re cipes-67012.

"Salmon & Asparagus with Lemon-Garlic Butter Sauce." 2023. EatingWell. https://www.eatingwell.com/recipe/262919/salmon-asparagus-with-lemon-ga rlic-butter-sauce/.

Saripalli, Vara. 2022. "15 Benefits of Journaling and Tips for Getting Started." Healthline. February 22, 2022. https://www.healthline.com/health/benefits-of-journaling.

Scarlett, Cathy. 2023. "11 Lifestyle Changes for Improving Mental Health." Afpafitness.

https://www.afpafitness.com/blog/11-lifestyle-changes-that-will-boost-your-m ental-health.

Scott, Jane. 2019. "Nana's Gluten Free Lemon Blueberry Muffins." Mom Loves Baking. October 23, 2019. https://www.momlovesbaking.com/nanas-gluten-free-lemon-blueberry-muffin s/.

"Sheet-Pan Roasted Root Vegetables." 2023. EatingWell. https://www.eatingwell.com/recipe/257723/sheet-pan-roasted-root-vegetables/.

"SIBO: Symptoms, Causes, Treatment, and Diet." 2019. Www.medicalnewstoday.com. February 19, 2019. https://www.medicalnewsto day.com/articles/324475.

Sims, Maddy. 2022. "What Gut Health Experts *Really* Think about Those Gut Health Hacks on TikTok." HUM Nutrition Blog. October 18, 2022. https://www.humnutrition.com/blog/gut-health-hacks/.

Sorrenti, Vincenzo, Sawan Ali, Laura Mancin, Sergio Davinelli, Antonio Paoli, and Giovanni Scapagnini. 2020. "Cocoa Polyphenols and Gut Microbiota Interplay: Bioavailability, Prebiotic Effect, and Impact on Human Health." Nutrients 12 (7): 1908. https://doi.org/10.3390/nu12071908.

Spector, Nicole. 2018. "The Science behind Being 'Hangry.'" NBC News. July 2, 2018. https://www.nbcnews.com/better/pop-culture/science-behind-being-hangry-n cna887806.

"Spicy Lentil Soup." 2023. Allrecipes. https://www.allrecipes.com/recipe/220391/spicy-lentil-soup/.

"Stress Relieving Journal Prompts." 2023.Northwestern State University. https://www.nsula.edu/stress-relieving-journal-prompts/.

Stutter Health. 2019. "Eating Well for Mental Health | Sutter Health." Sutterhealth.org. 2019. https://www.sutterhealth.org/health/nutri tion/eating-well-for-mental-health.

Surprising Reasons You're Gaining Weight." WebMD. 2019. https://www.webmd.com/diet/ss/slideshow-weight-gain-shockers.

Tang, W. 2022. 15 Gut Health Hacks for a Healthier You. Best in Nature. December 16 2022. https://www.bestinnature.com/blog/post/gut-health-hacks

"The Estrobolome: A Bridge between Gut Health and Hormonal

Balance | Blog." 2023. Www.lencolab.com. https://www.lencolab.-com/publications/2021/12/the-estrobolome-a-bridge-be tween-gut.html.

"The Estrobolome: How Microbes Affect Estrogen Metabolism & Cancer Risk." 2018. Holistic Primary Care. August 7, 2018. https://holisticprimarycare.net/topics/cancer-care/the-estrobolome-how-micr obes-affect-estrogen-metabolism-cancer-risk/.

"The GI Diet - List of Low GI Foods." 2023. Www.the-Gi-Diet.org. https://www.the-gi-diet.org/lowgifoods/.

"The Gut-Brain Connection: How It Works and the Role of Nutrition." 2018. Healthline. June 27, 2018. https://www.healthline.com/nutrition/gut-brain-connection#TOC_TITLE_H DR_3.

"The Gut Microbiome and Brain Health - Memory and Brain Wellness Center." 2023. Depts.washington.edu. https://depts.washington.e-du/mbwc/news/article/the-gut-microbiome-and-br ain-health.

"The Link between Gut Health & Hormones Explained | the Nutrition Professionals." 2023. https://nutritionpro.net/the-link-between-gut-health-hormones-explained/.

"The Microbiome." The Nutrition Source. August 16, 2017. https://www.hsph.harvard.edu/nutritionsource/microbiome/#mi-crobiota-ben efit.

"The Vagus Nerve: Your Key to Managing IBS." 2023. Www.mind-sethealth.com. https://www.mindsethealth.com/matter/vagus-nerve-ibs.

"These Simple Exercises Can Improve Your Digestive Health and Melt Your Belly Fat Quickly!" 2023. NDTV.com. https://www.ndtv.com/health/these-simple-exercises-can-improve-your-digestive-health-and-melt-your-belly-fat-quickly-1995184.

"Tomato and Leek Frittata with Goat Cheese." 2023. Martha Stewart. Accessed May 2, 2023. https://www.marthastewart.com/1154581/tomato-and-leek-frittata.

Tooley, Katie Louise. 2020. "Effects of the Human Gut Microbiota on Cognitive Performance, Brain Structure and Function: A Narrative

Review." Nutrients 12 (10): 3009. https://doi.org/10.3390/nu12103009.

Tucker, Alexa. 2018. "5 Essential Calf Stretches Everyone Should Be Doing." SELF. https://www.self.com/gallery/essential-calf-stretches.

Tucker, Alexa. 2023. "How to Start Working out If You've Never Exercised Before." SELF. https://www.self.com/story/steps-to-take-start-working-out-for-first-time.

"Vegan Buddha Bowl." 2020. Loving It Vegan. July 27, 2020. https://lovingitvegan.com/vegan-buddha-bowl/.

Wang, Hao, Chuan-Xian Wei, Lu Min, and Ling-Yun Zhu. 2018. "Good or Bad: Gut Bacteria in Human Health and Diseases." Biotechnology & Biotechnological Equipment 32 (5): 1075–80. https://doi.org/10.1080/13102818.2018.1481350.

"Warm Brown Rice and Chicken Salad." 2023. Healthy Food Guide. Accessed April 26, 2023. https://www.healthyfood.com/healthy-recipes/warm-brown-rice-and-chickensalad/.

Warren, Miriam Frankel and Matt. 2023. "How Gut Bacteria Are Controlling Your Brain." Www.bbc.com. https://www.bbc.com/future/article/20230120-how-gut-bacteria-are-controlling-your-brain.

"What Causes Dysbiosis and How Is It Treated?" 2017. Healthline. September 19, 2017. https://www.healthline.com/health/digestive-health/dysbiosis#prevention.

What is a Telomere? 2009. T.A. Sciences®. 2009. https://www.tasciences.com/what-is-a-telomere.html.

"What Is Healthy Aging?" 2023. Www.nutritionnews.abbott. https://www.nutritionnews.abbott/healthy-living/aging-well/What-Is-Healthy -Aging-/.

Yeagle, P. 2015. "Microbiome of Uncontacted Amerindians." Science 348 (6232): 298–98. https://doi.org/10.1126/science.348.6232.298-a.

"Yes, You Can Exercise When You Have Literally No Time—Here's How to Hack Your Fitness Routine." 2023. EatingWell. Accessed

April 14, 2023.https://www.eatingwell.com/article/7833111/exercise-when-you-have-no-time/.

Zhang, Yu-Jie, Sha Li, Ren-You Gan, Tong Zhou, Dong-Ping Xu, and Hua-Bin Li. 2015. "Impacts of Gut Bacteria on Human Health and Diseases." International Journal of Molecular Sciences 16 (12): 7493–7519. https://doi.org/10.3390/ijms16047493.

Milton Keynes UK
Ingram Content Group UK Ltd.
UKHW030141120324
439192UK00011B/839

9 798224 437566